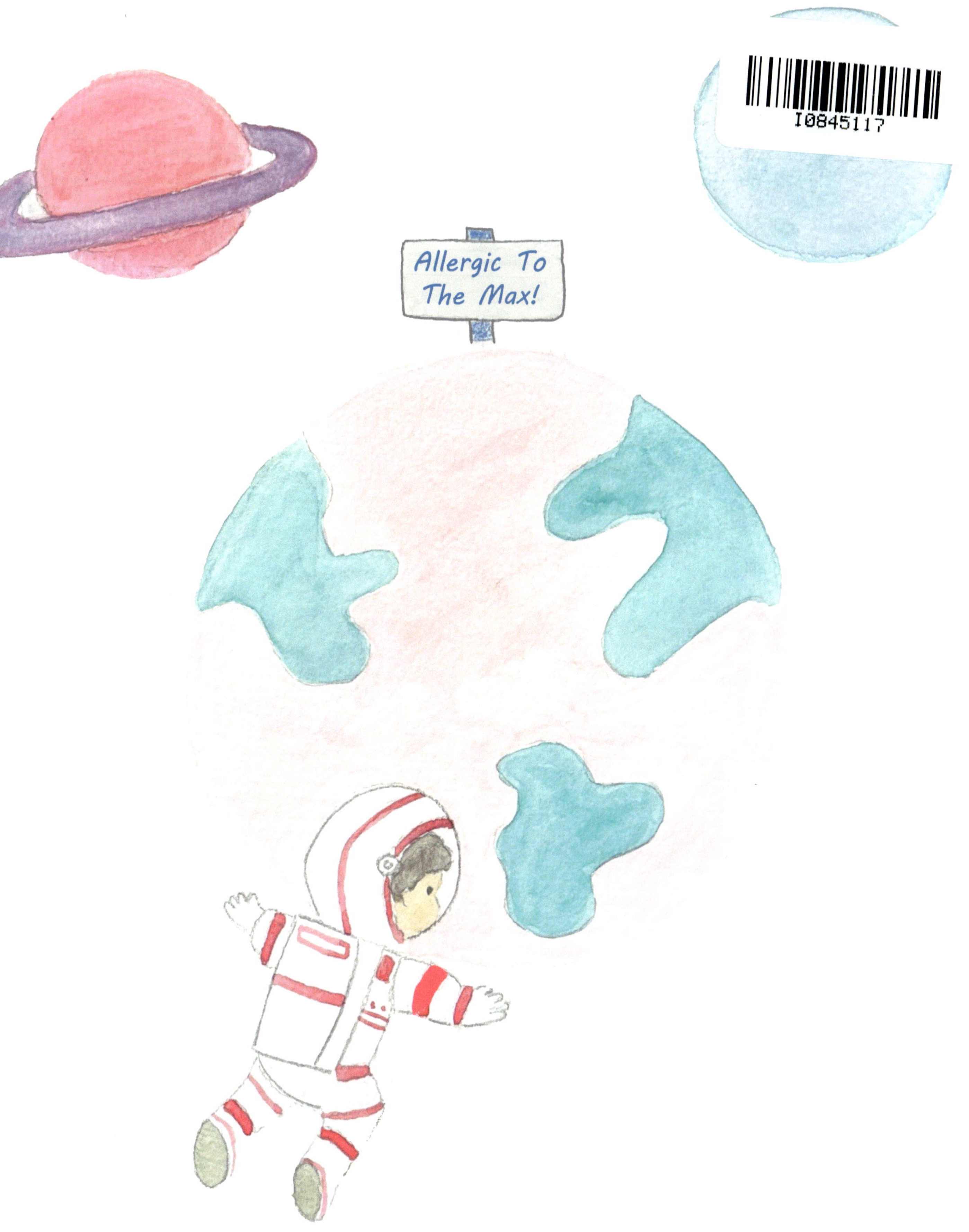

Allergic To The Max!
I0845117
Illustrated and Written by Maxwell Ngo
Project support by Aayush Iyer

ISBN: 979-8-9994896-0-9

Illustrations by: Maxwell Ngo

Book Cover by: Maxwell Ngo

For permission requests, contact allergictothemax@gmail.com

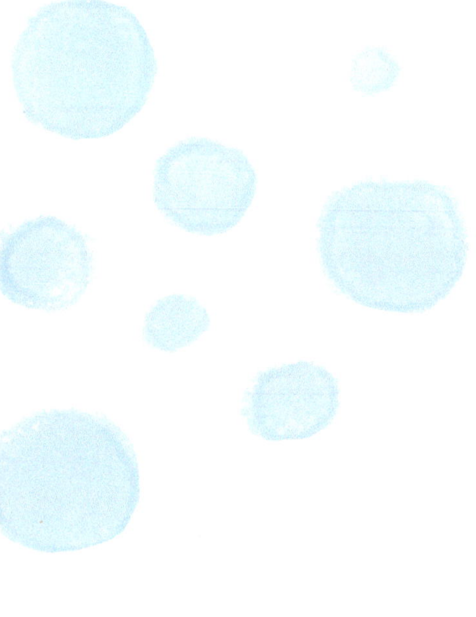

For my grandma and grandpa
- MN

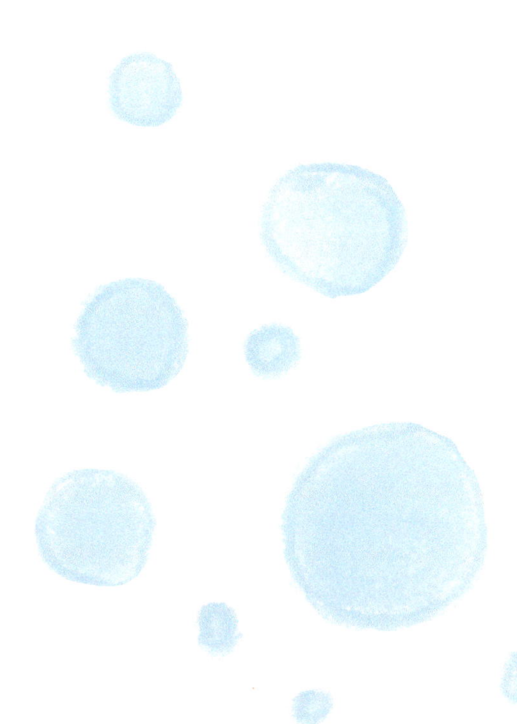

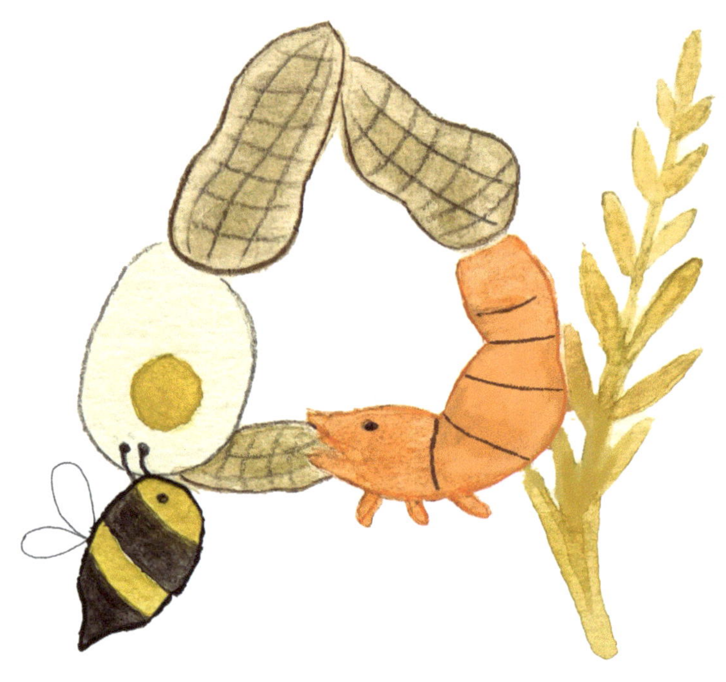

A is for Allergies.
They can make tummies upset.
Let's learn what they are
so we never forget!

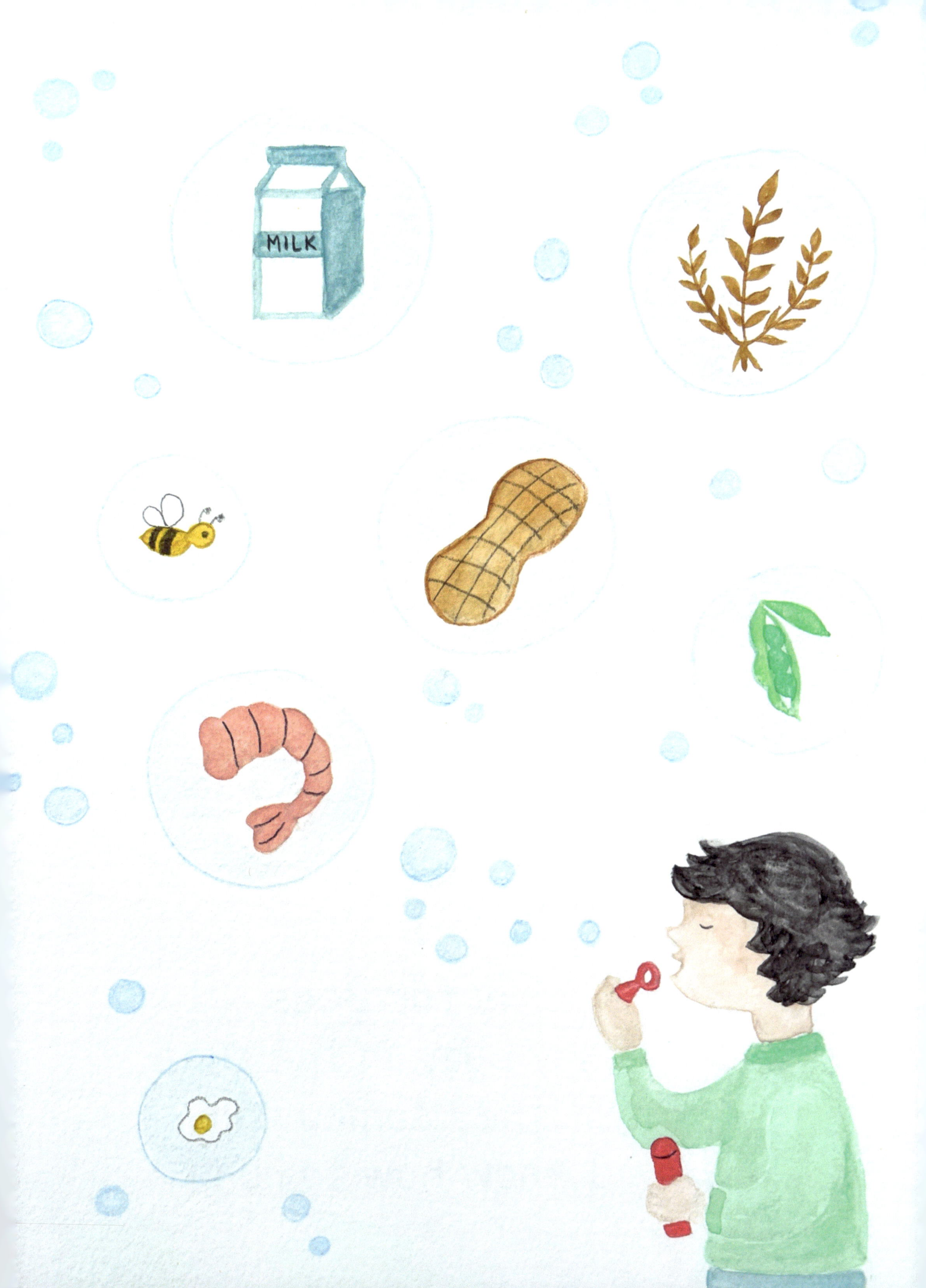

MILK

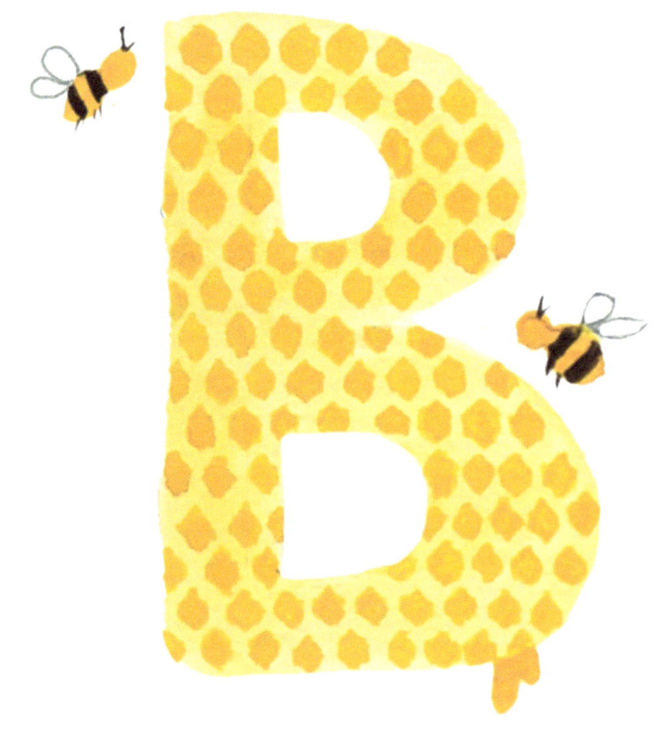

B is for Bees.
They buzz in the sun.
If they come near,
I know how to run.

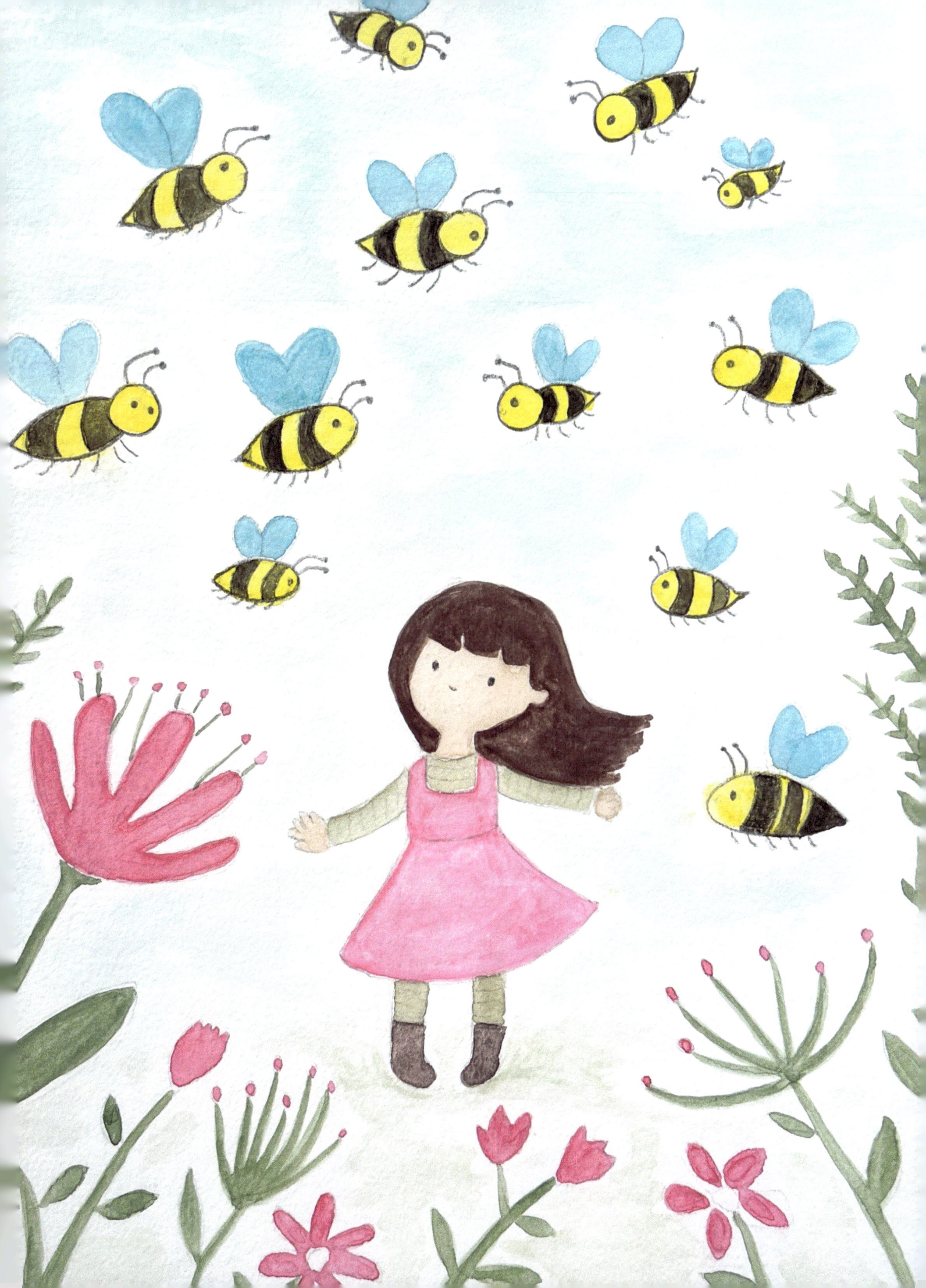

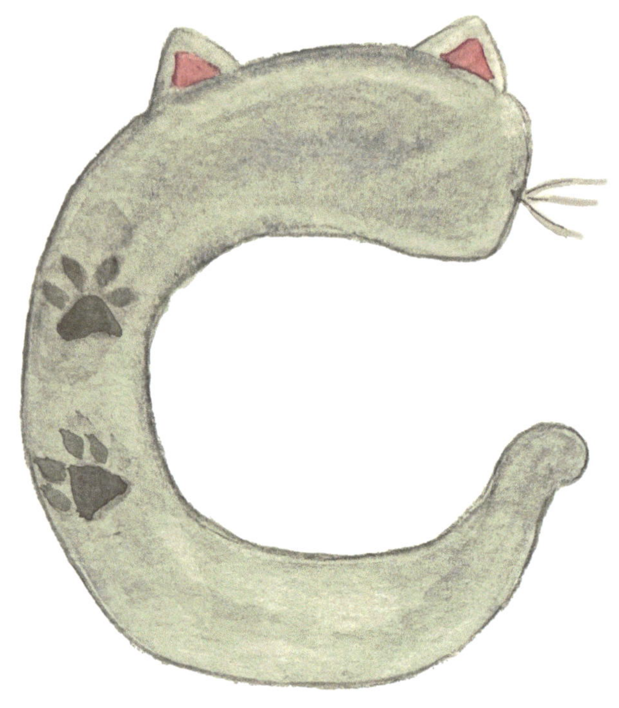

C is for Cats.
They are soft and sweet.
But their fur can make me
itchy from my head to my feet!

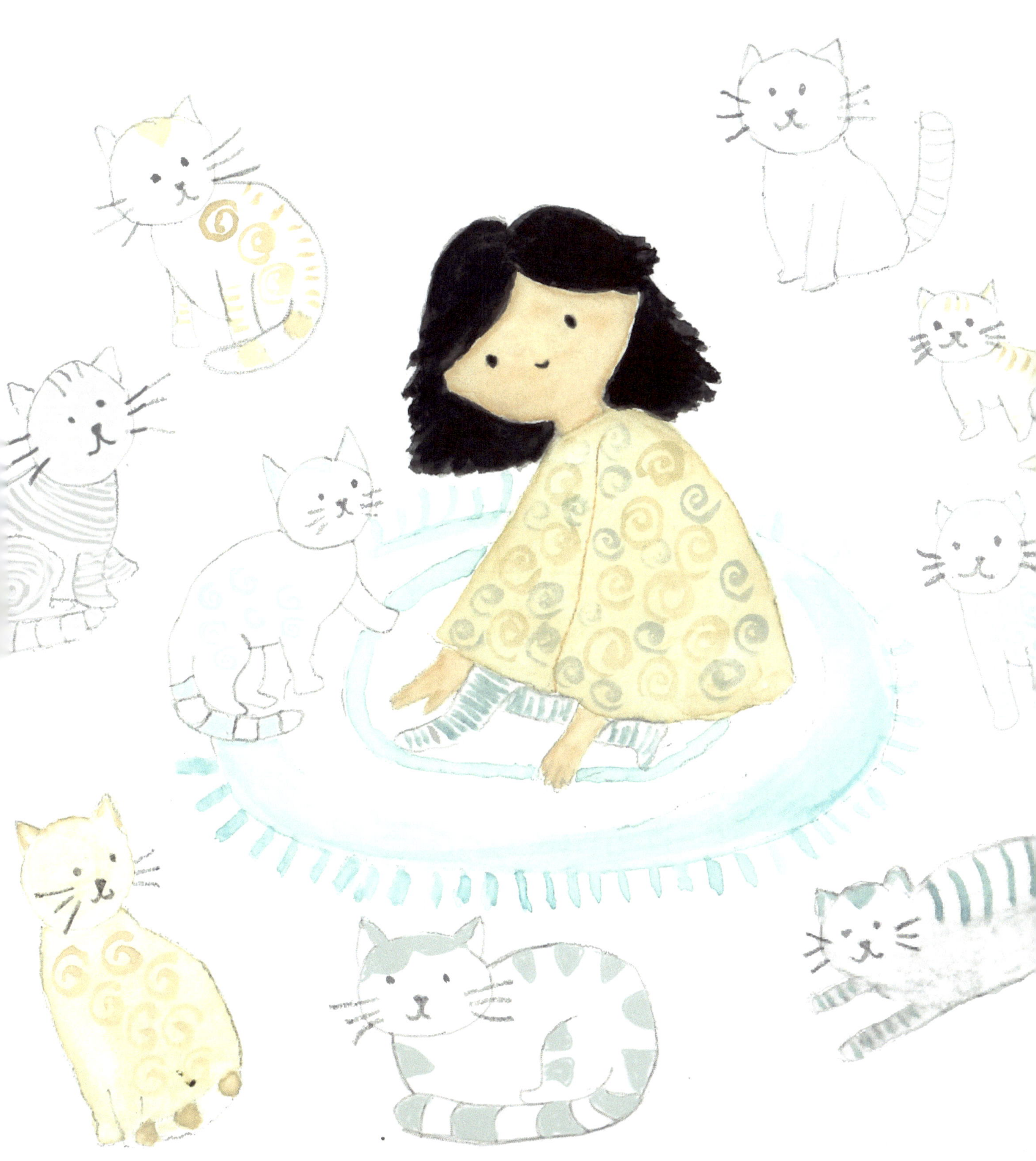

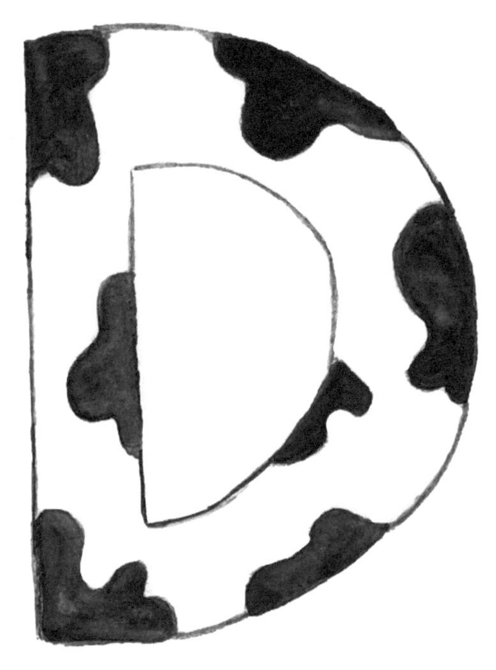

D is for Dairy.
Dairy is in milk and gooey cheese.
For some, they cause tummy
aches that won't ease.

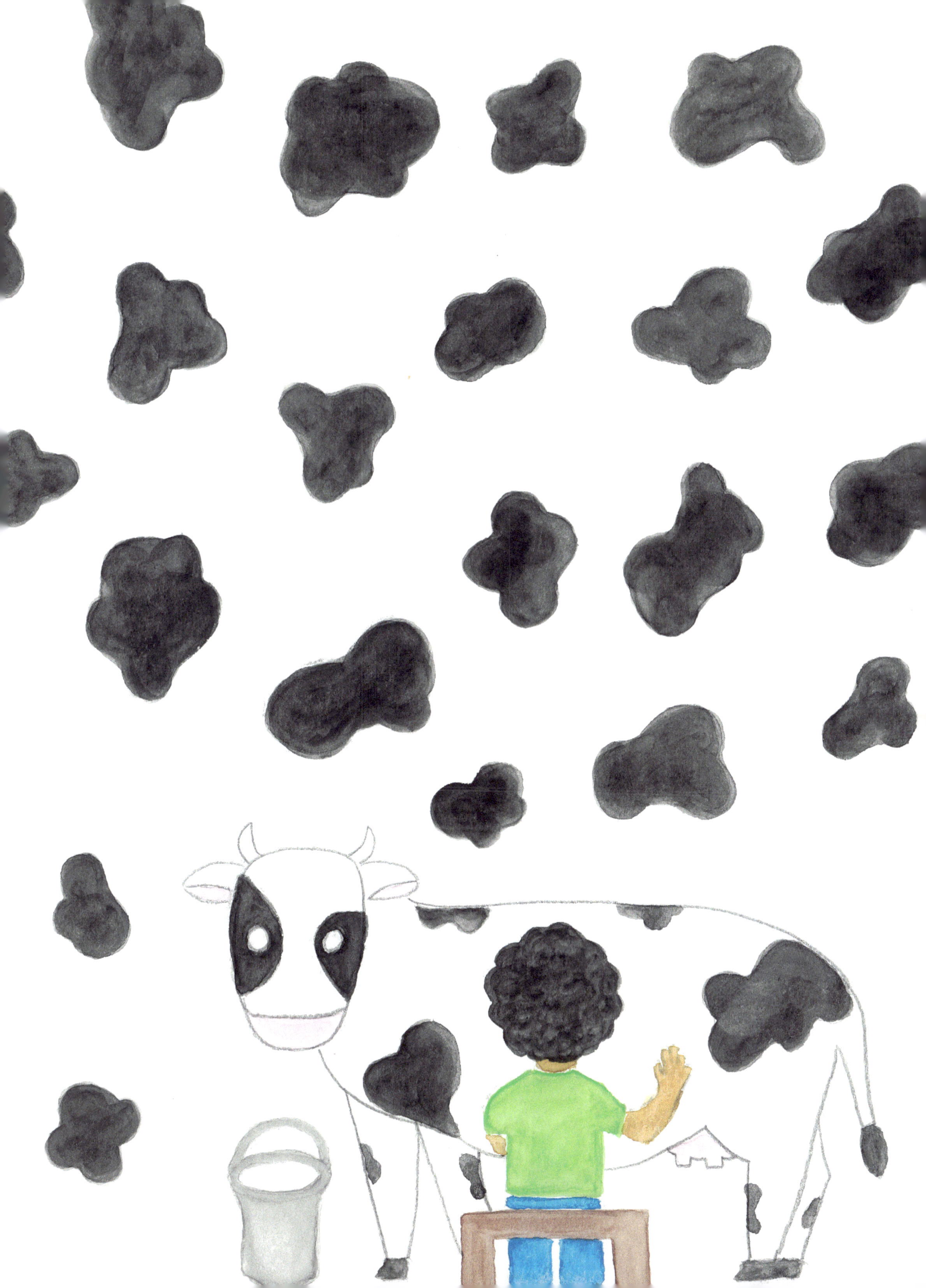

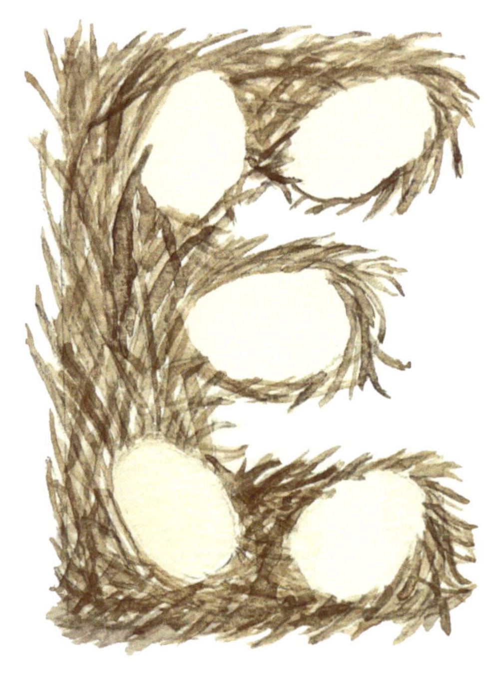

E is for eggs.
Some must beware,
as eggs are hidden in foods
found almost anywhere.

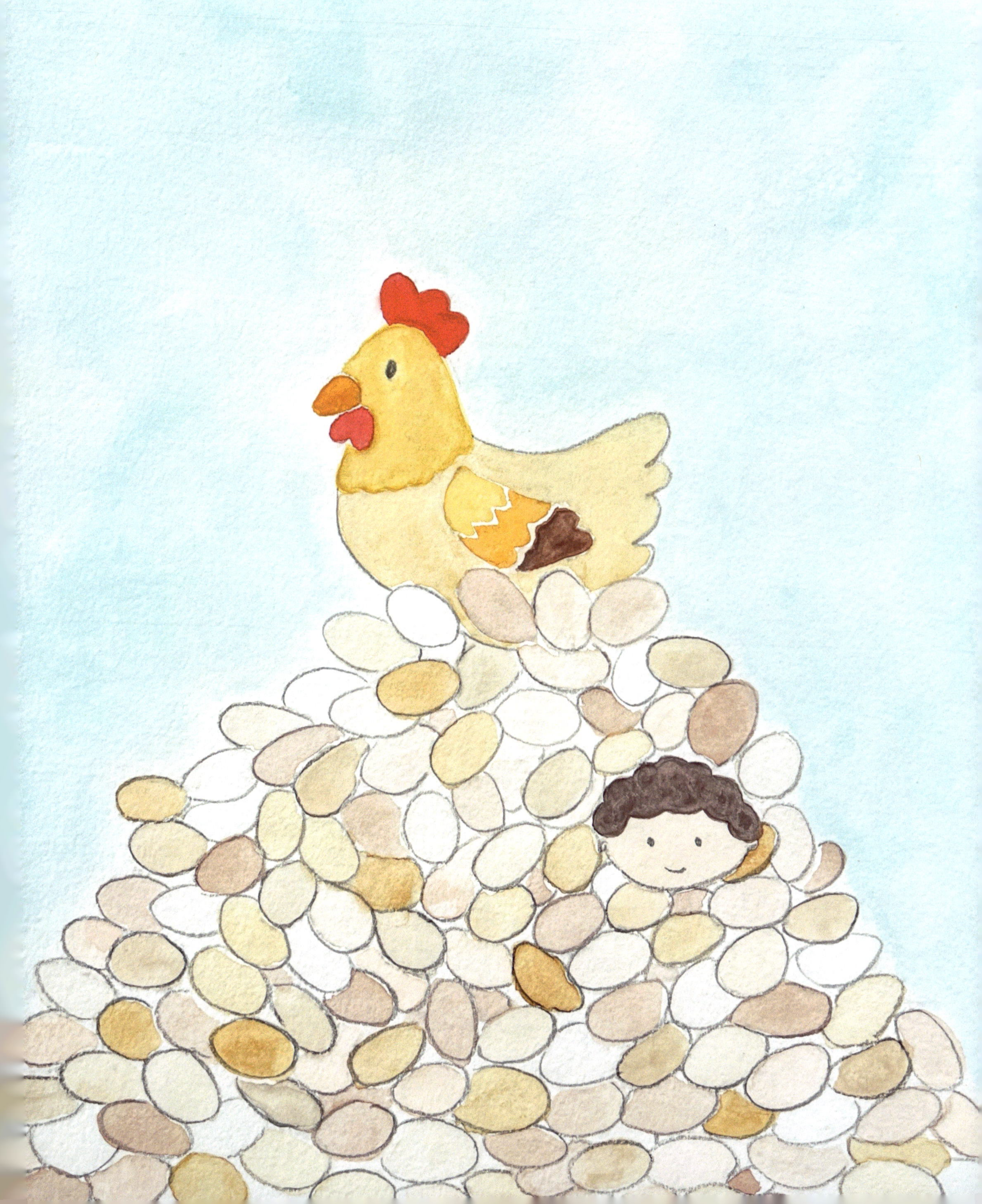

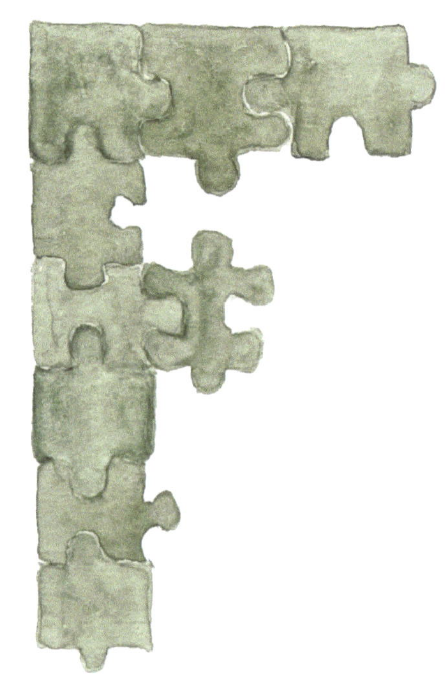

F is for Friends.
Friends help us each day.
They learn our needs and
keep danger away!

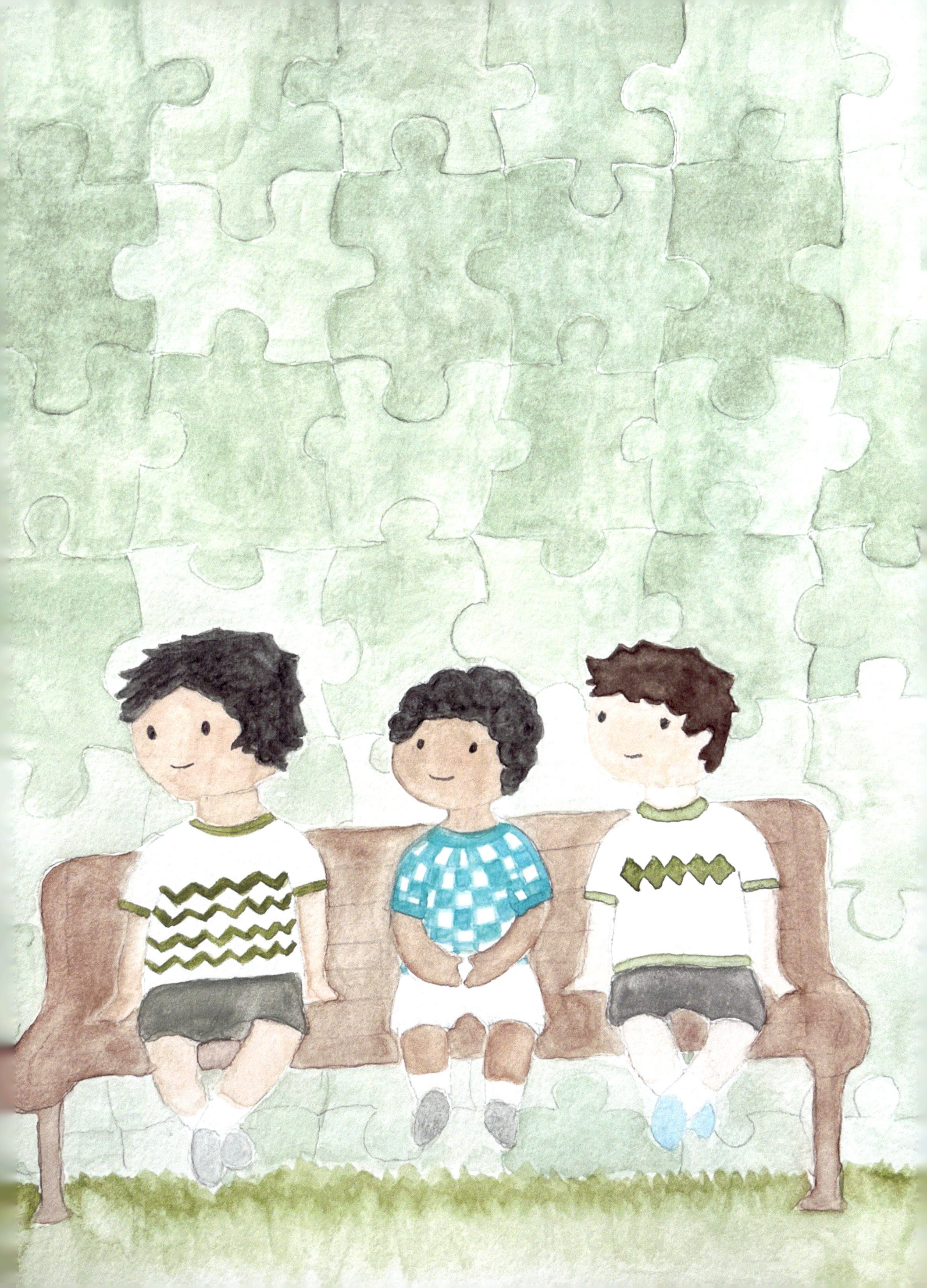

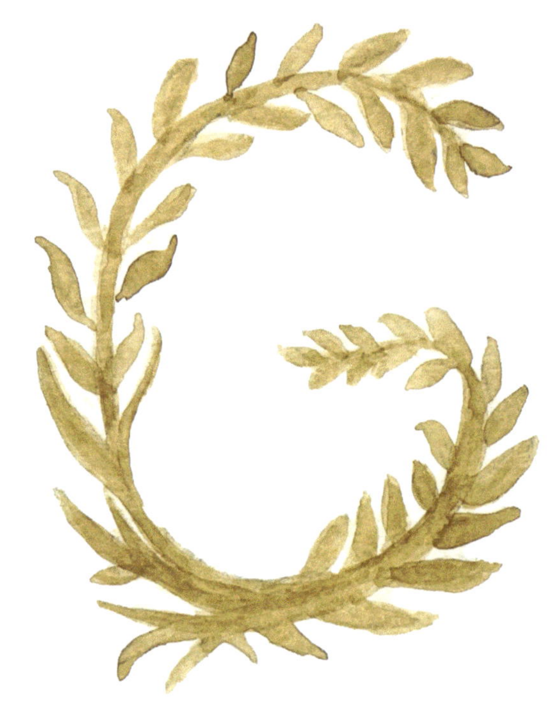

G is for Gluten-free.
Wheat, barley, and rye,
gluten-free goodies
are what I will try.

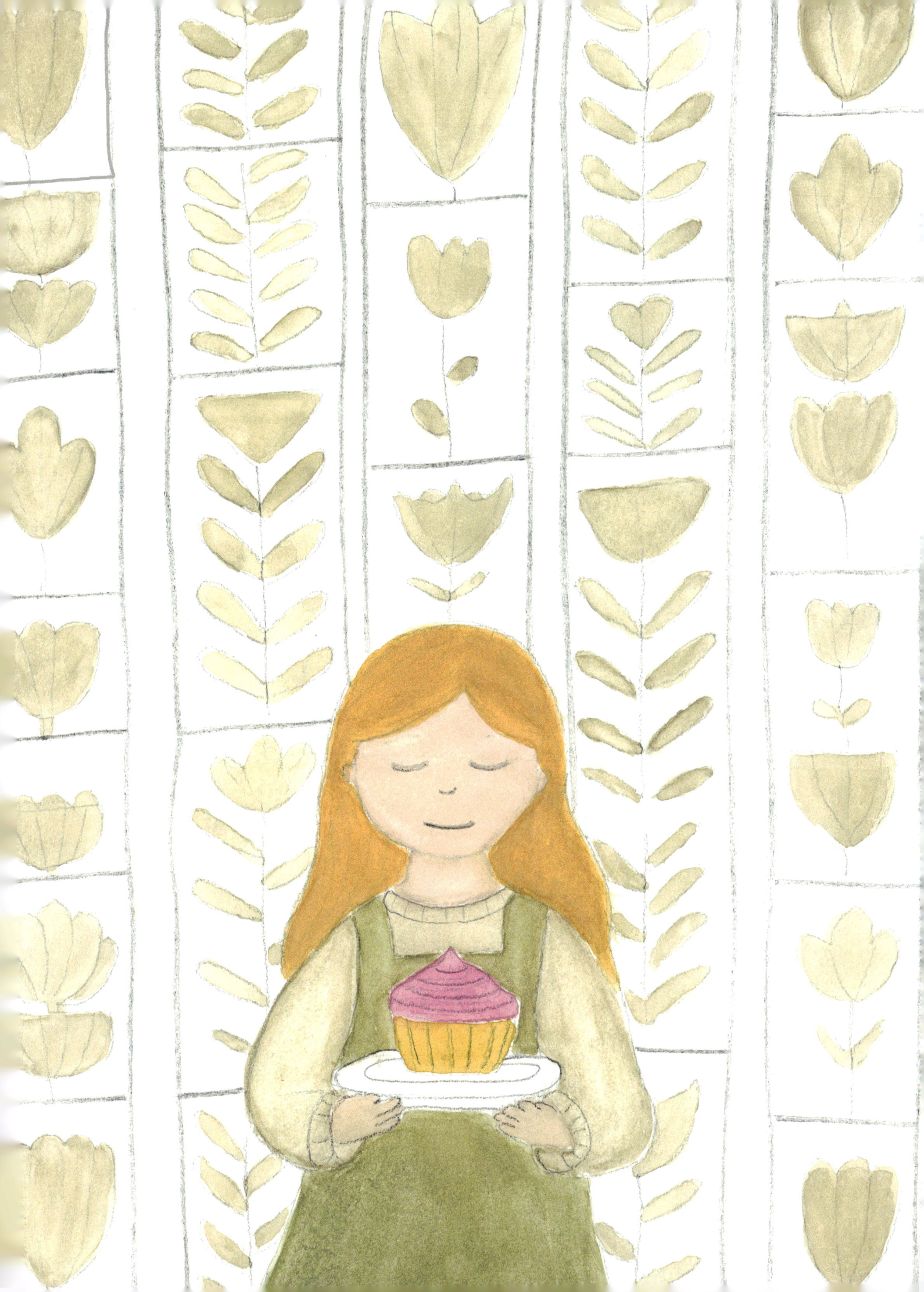

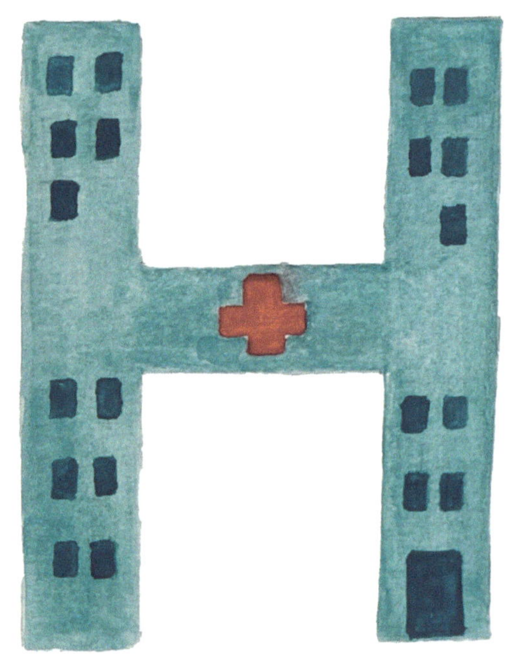

H is for Hospital.
They have doctors who care.
If a reaction starts,
they're always there.

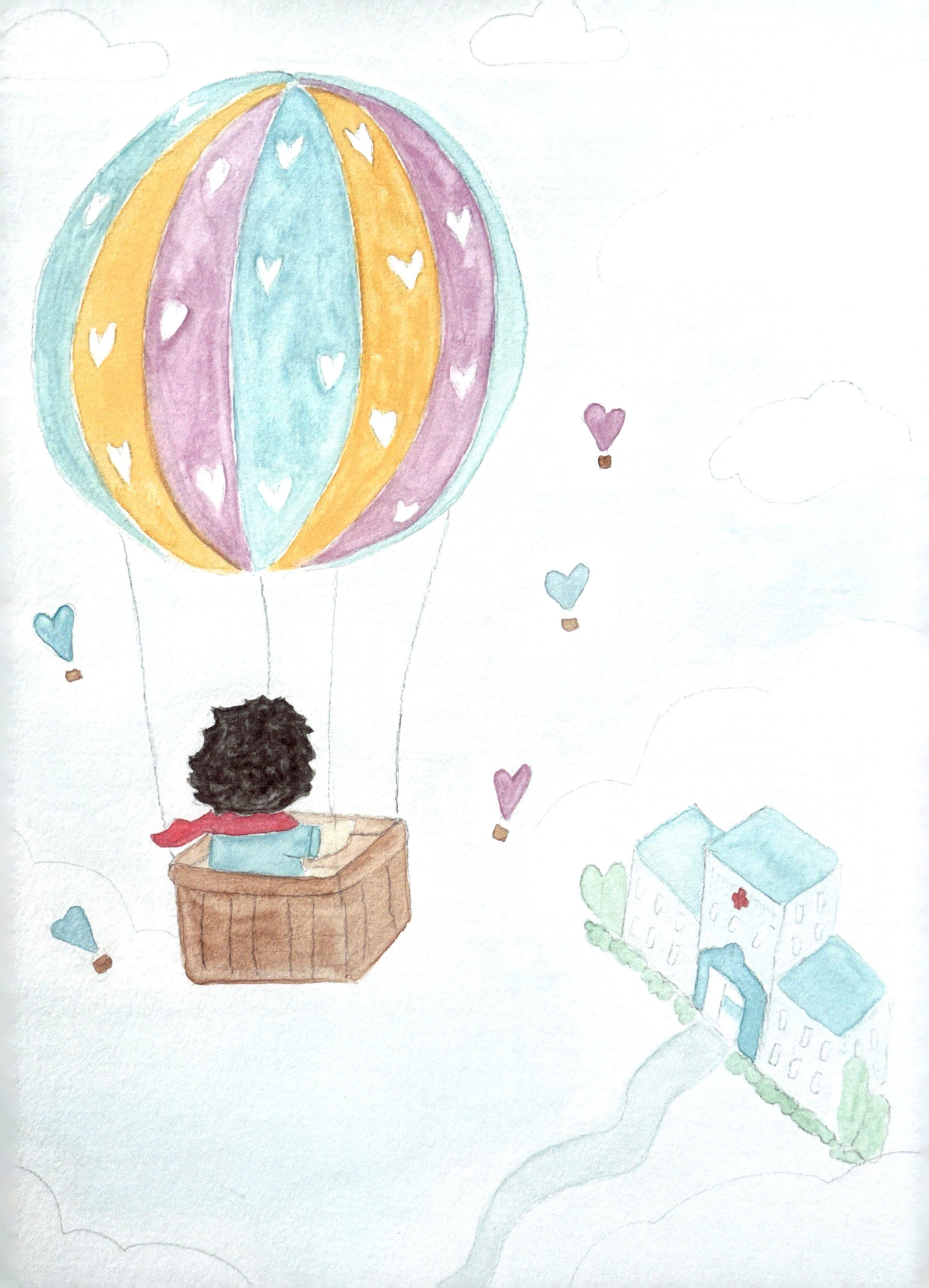

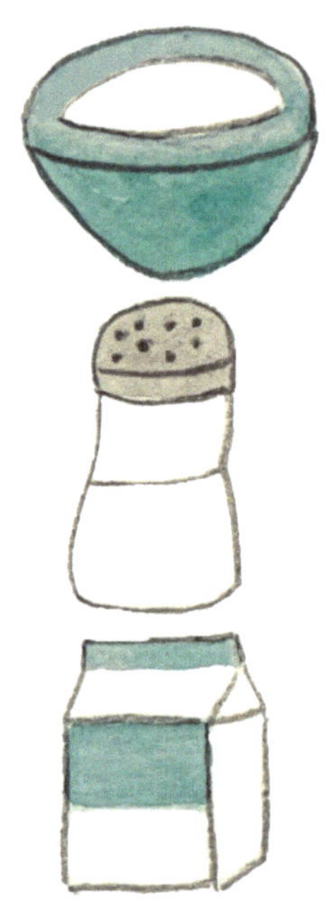

I is for Ingredients.
Check labels through and through.
It's the safest thing to do
before trying something new.

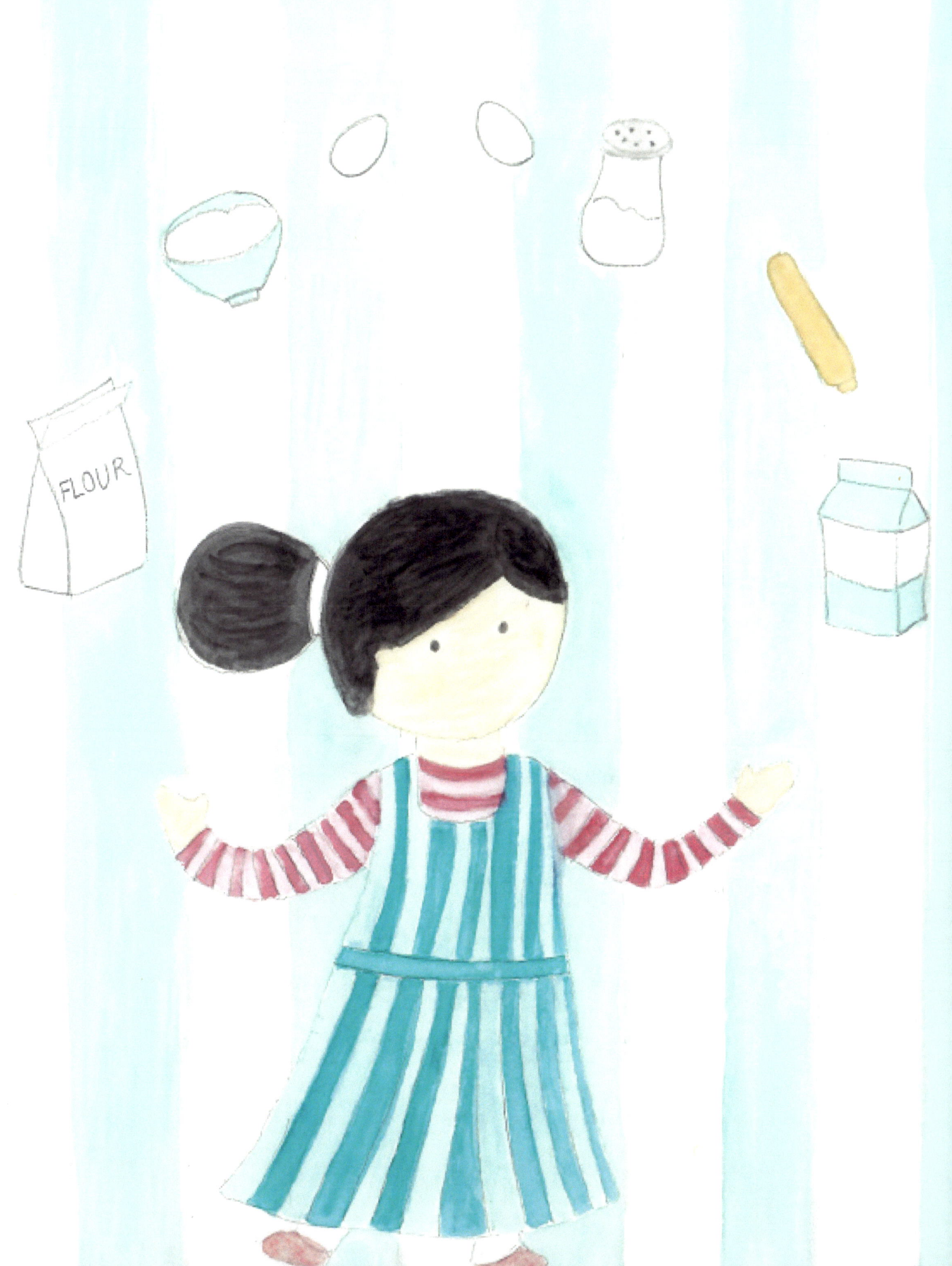

FLOUR

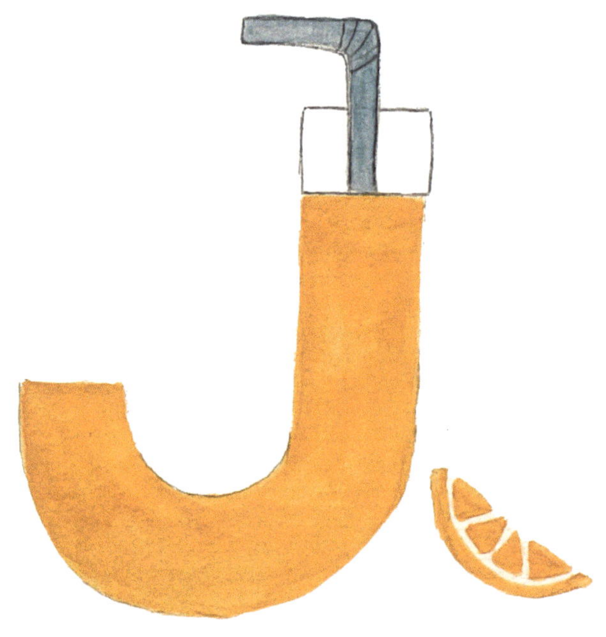

J is for Joy.
When my juice is just right,
no hidden surprises and
only fruity delight.

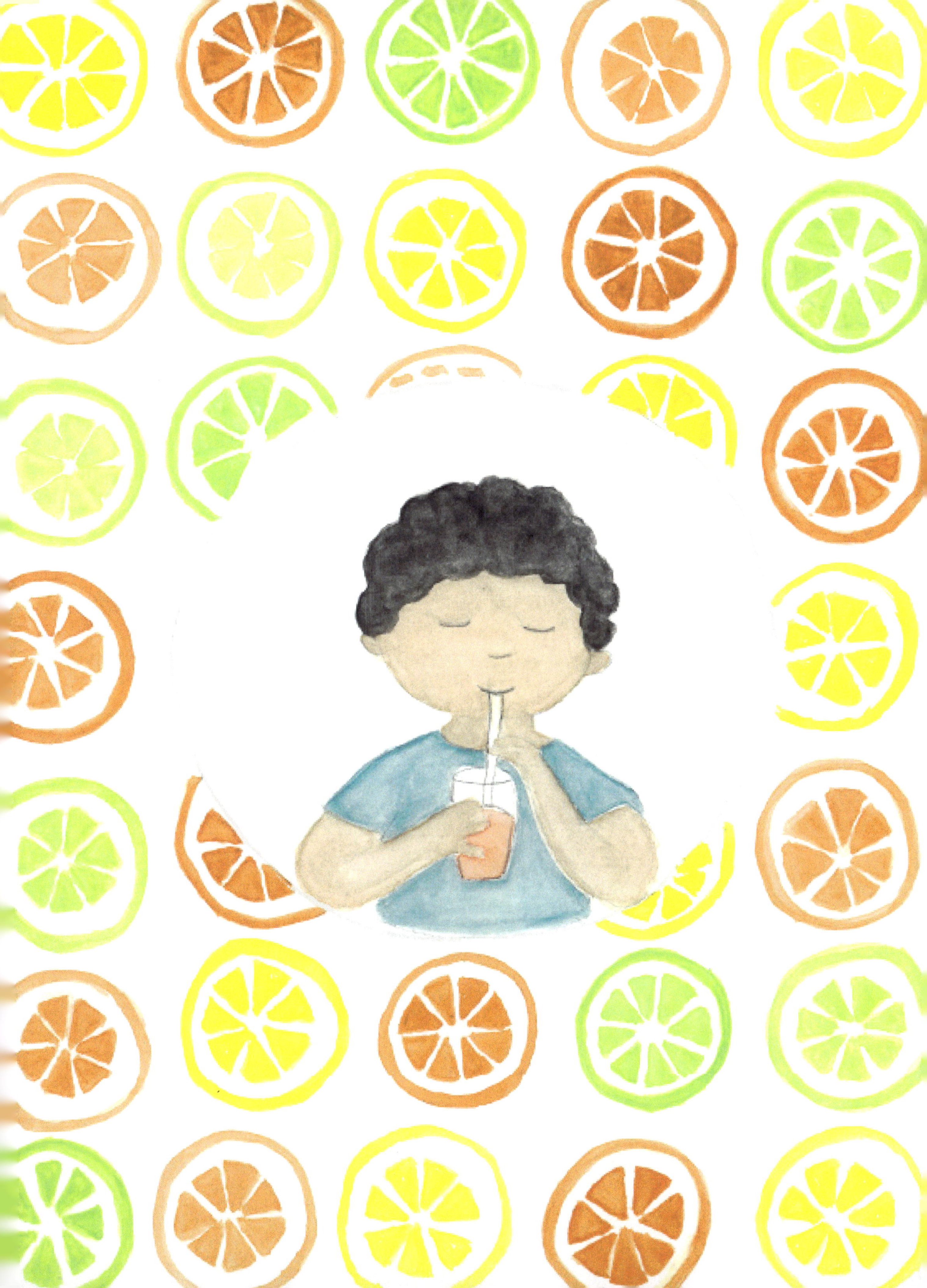

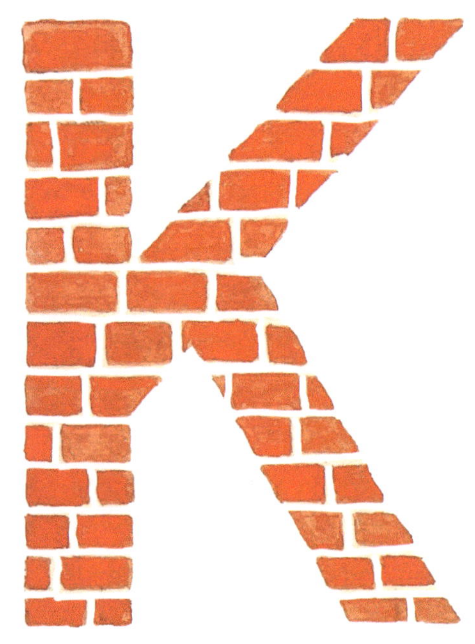

K is for Kindness.
It's shown in words and deeds,
from friends who ask questions
and help with allergy needs.

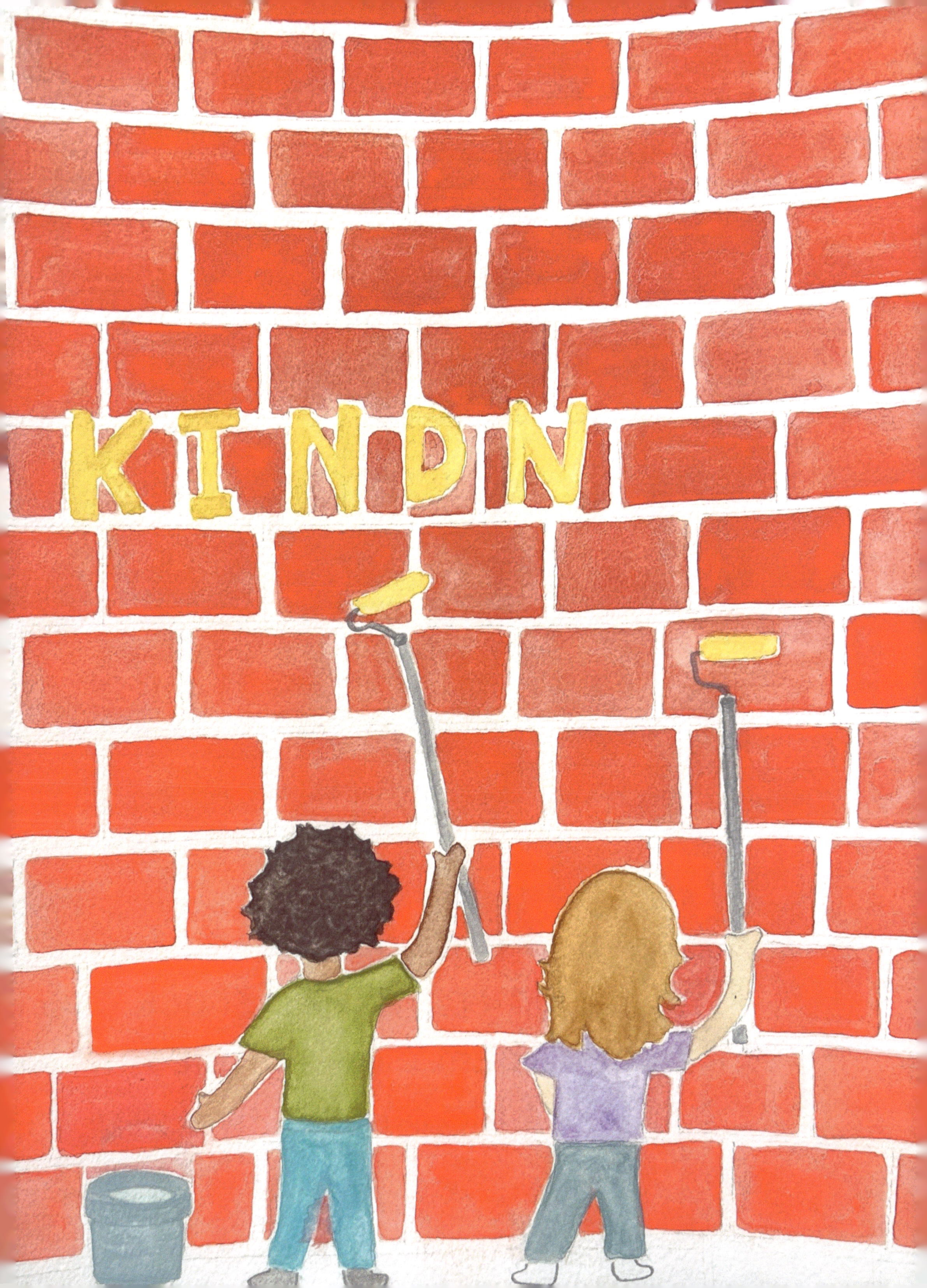
KINDN

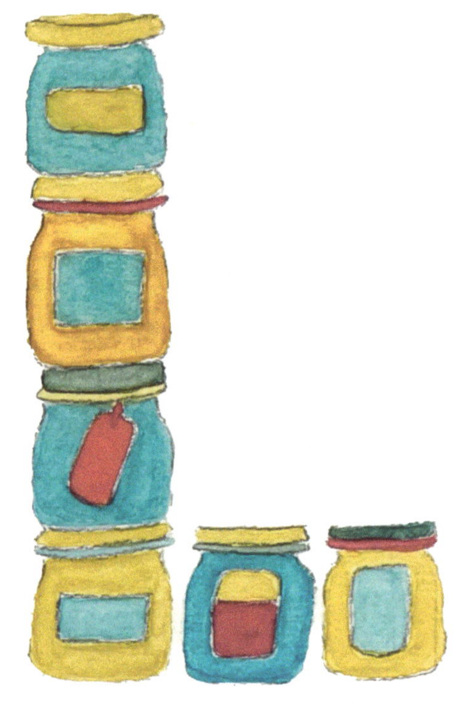

L is for Labels.
They're on each little snack.
Reading them closely helps
keep me on track!

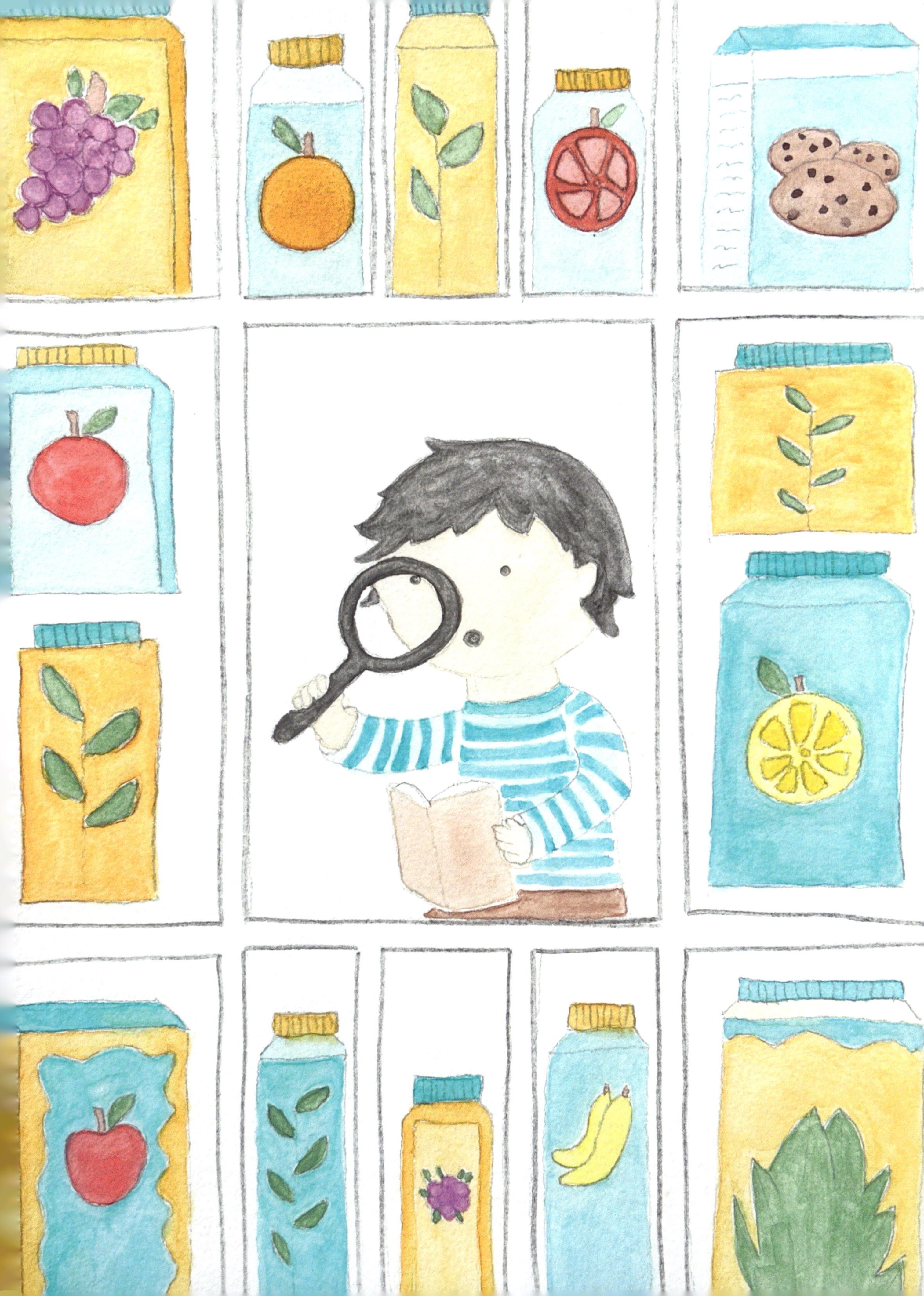

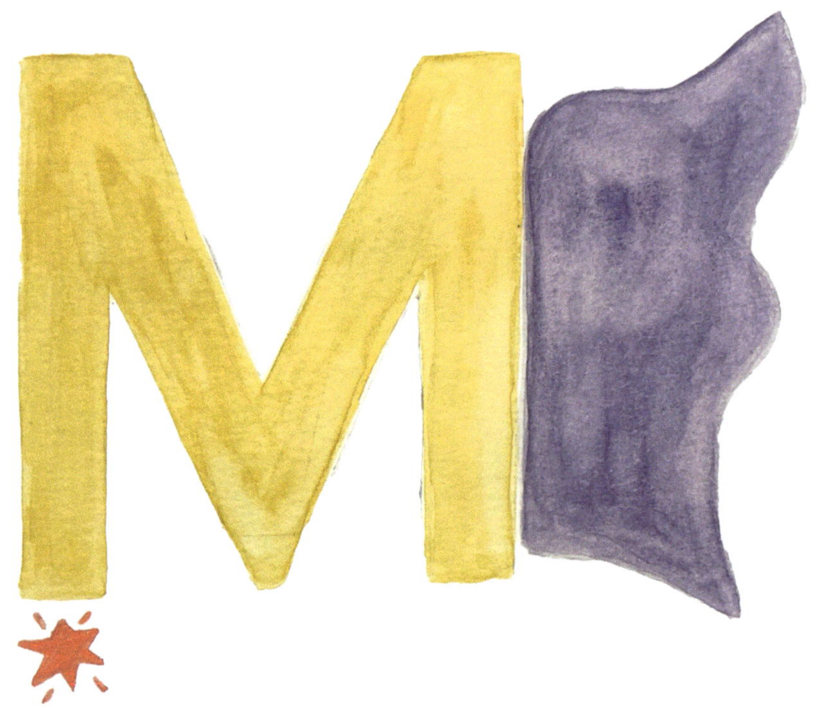

M is for Mighty.
I'm strong and I know
how to stay safe
wherever I go.

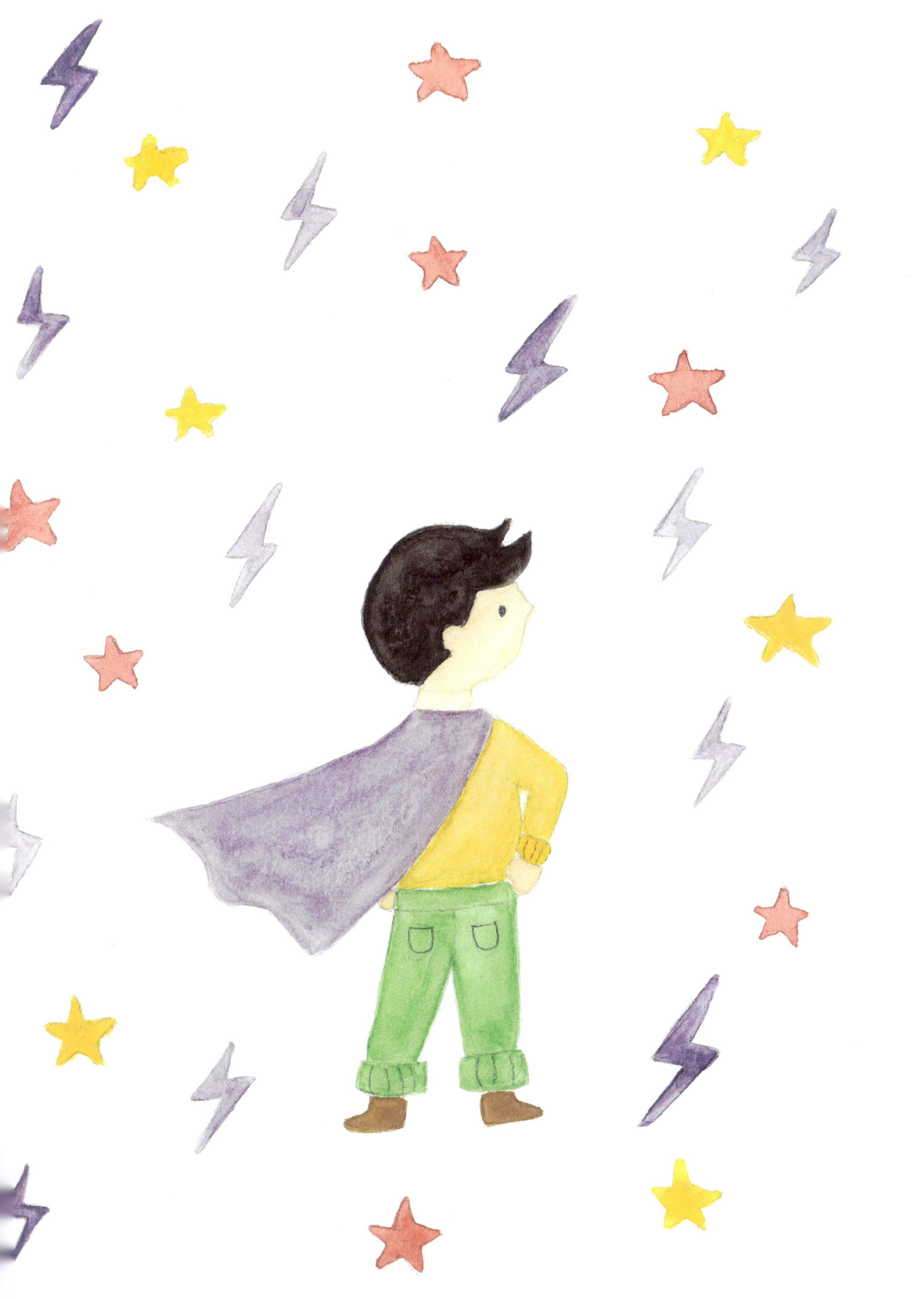

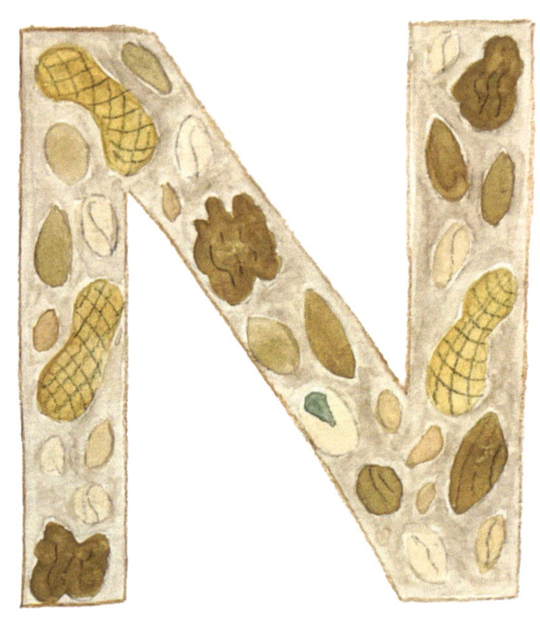

N is for Nuts.
Like almonds and more,
if I see them nearby
I head for the door.

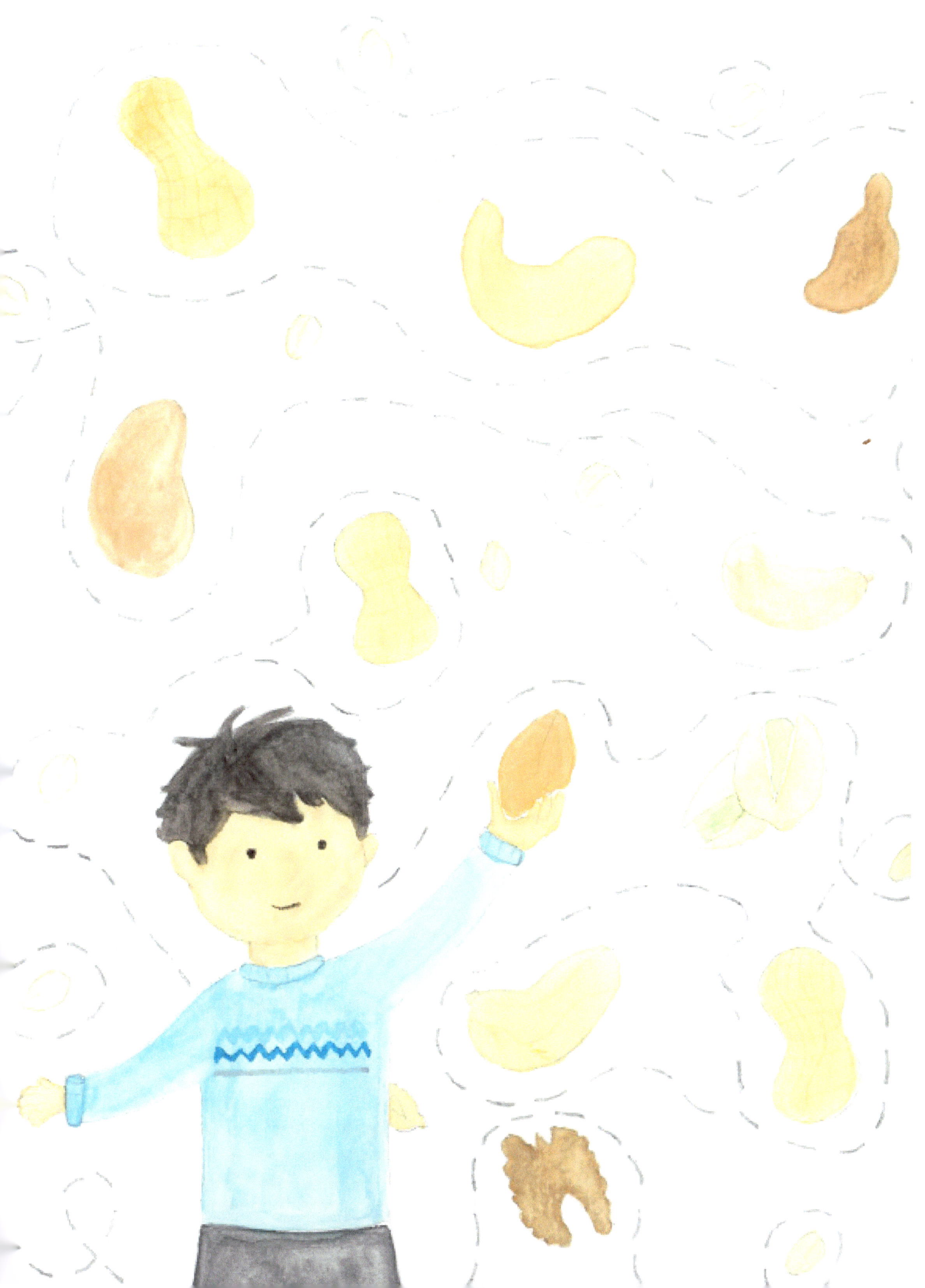

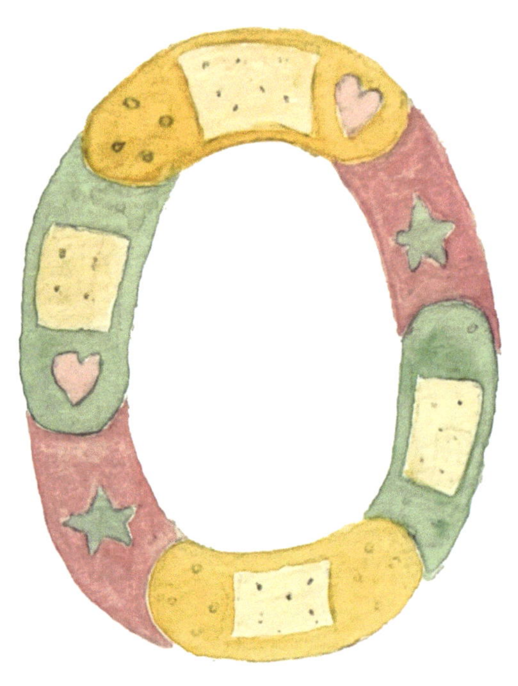

O is for Ouch!
When I get a red lump,
I know it's a sign,
not just a bump.

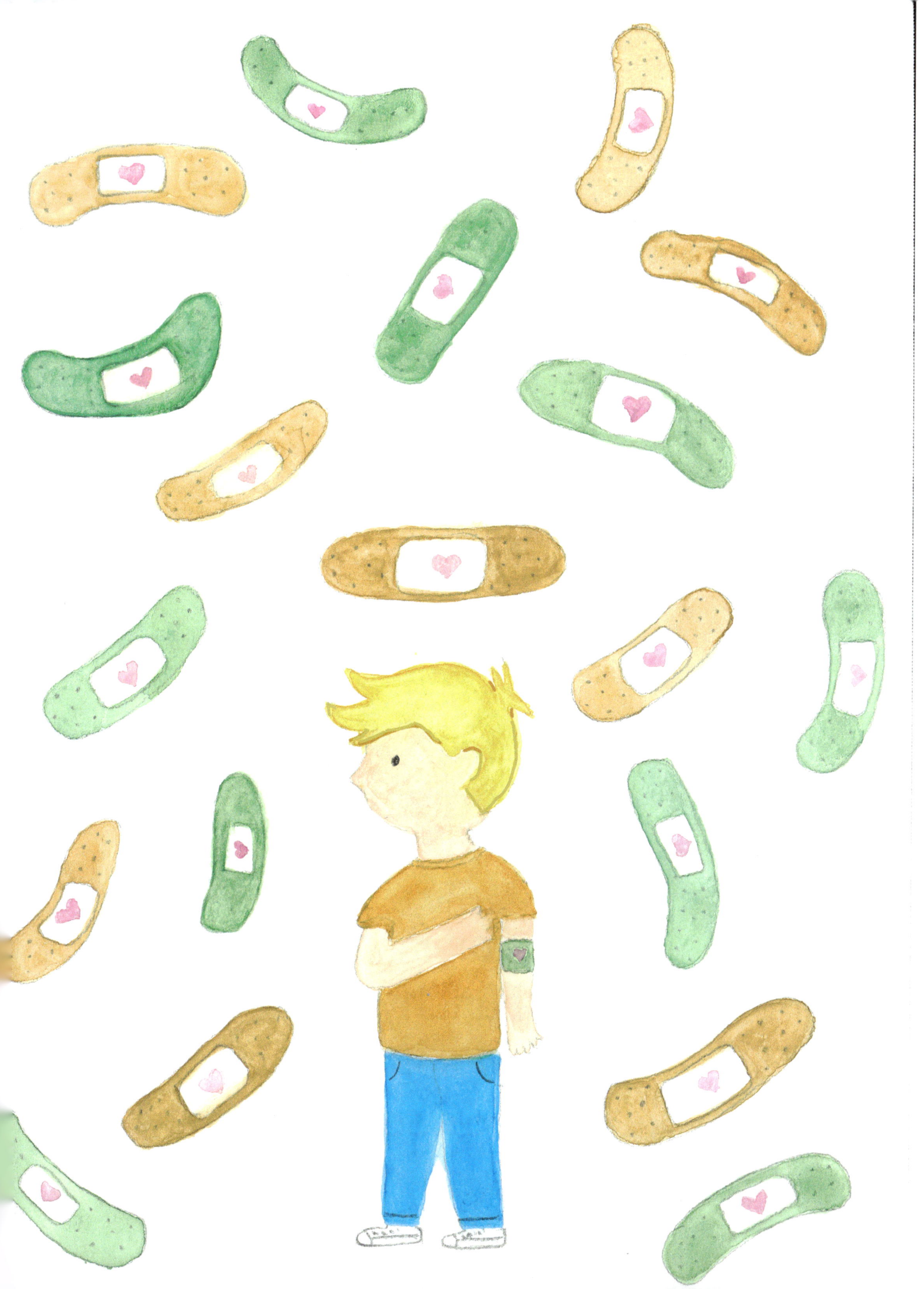

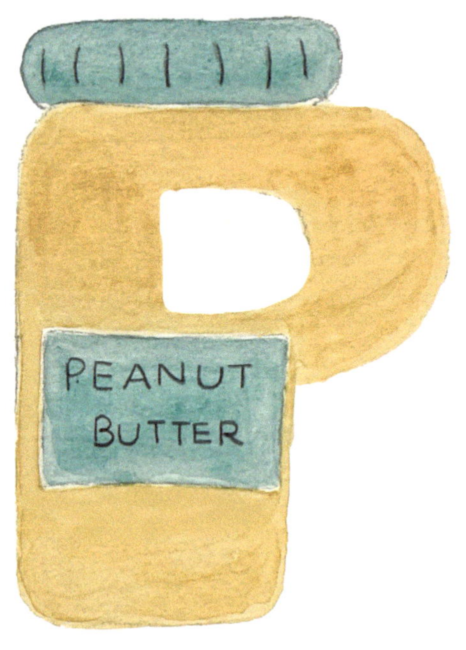

P is for Peanuts.
They're crunchy and sweet,
but for some kids,
they're not safe to eat.

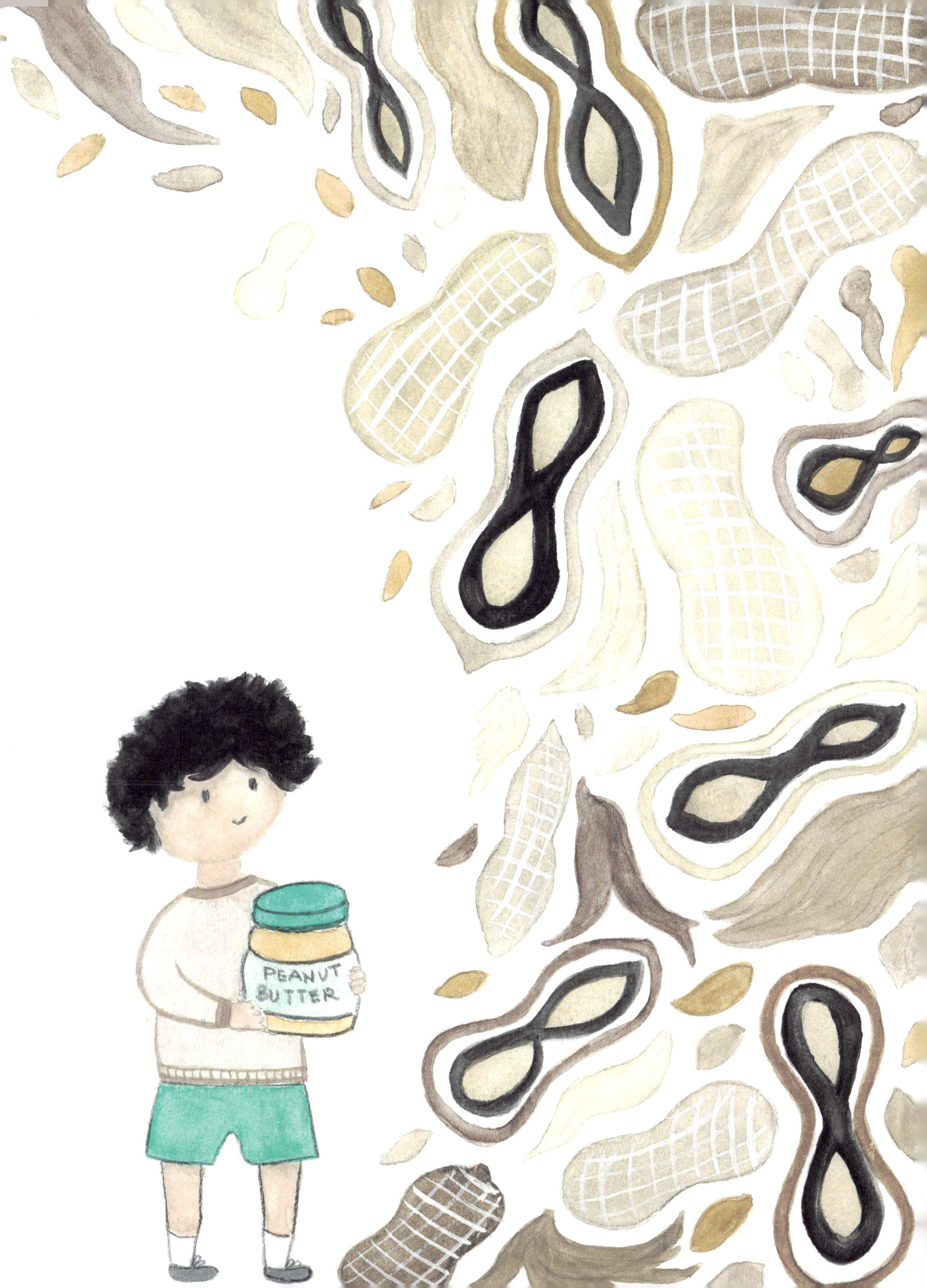
PEANUT
BUTTER

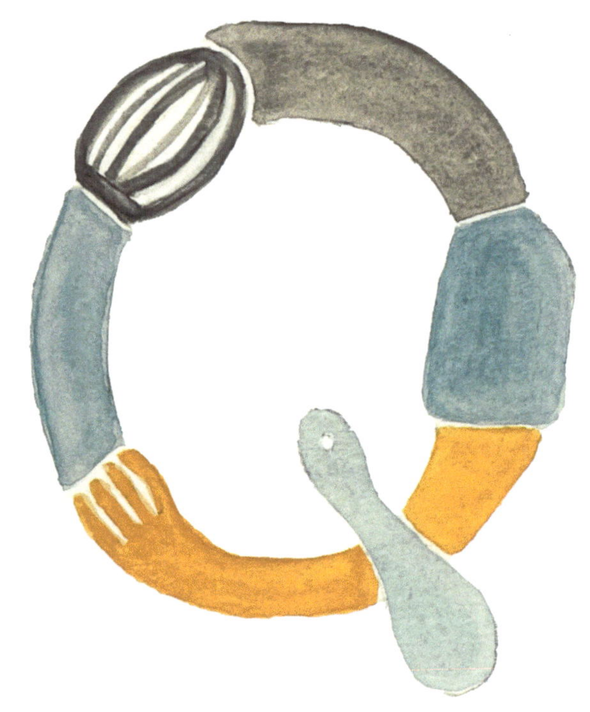

Q is for Questions.
Whether big or small,
asking them first helps
avoid a close call.

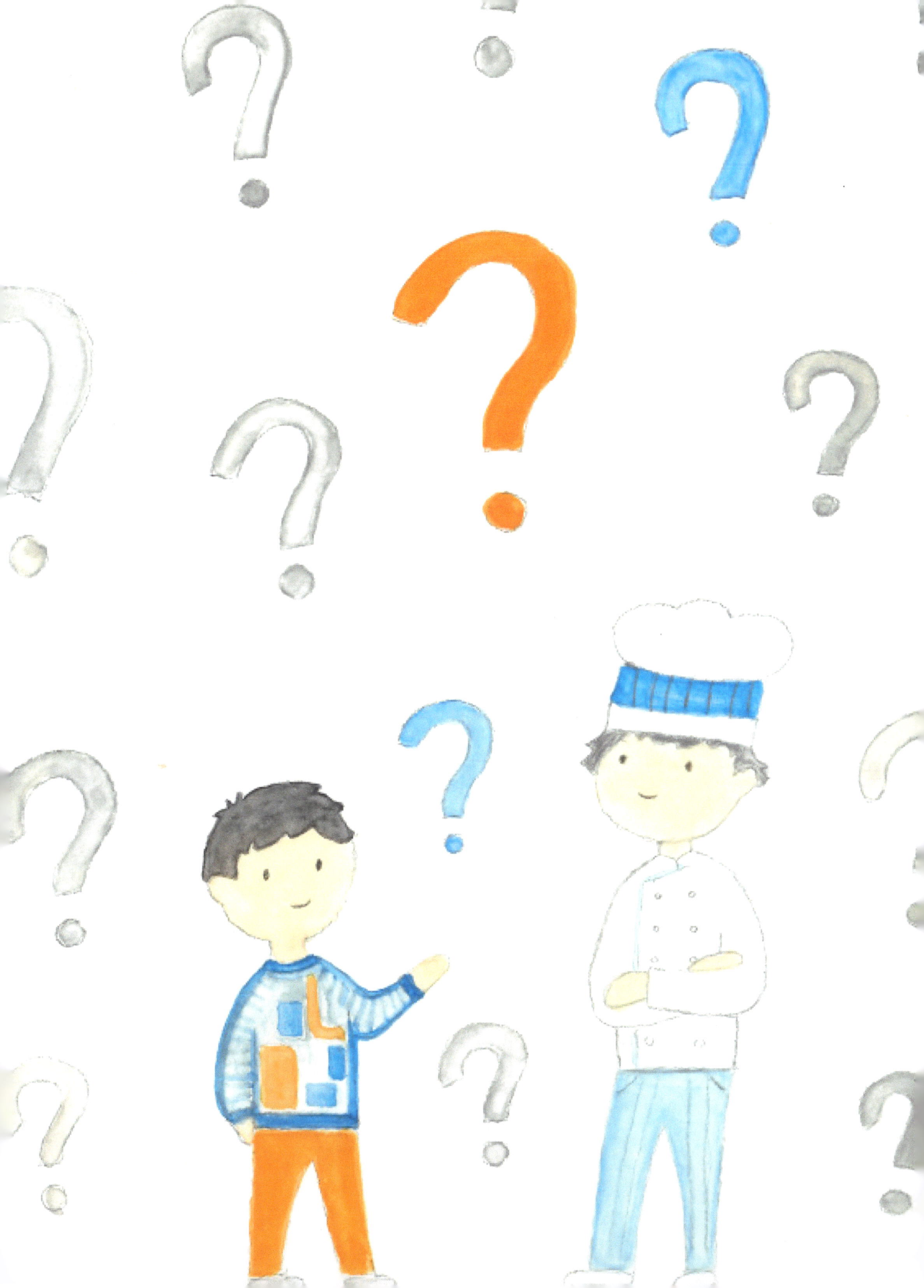

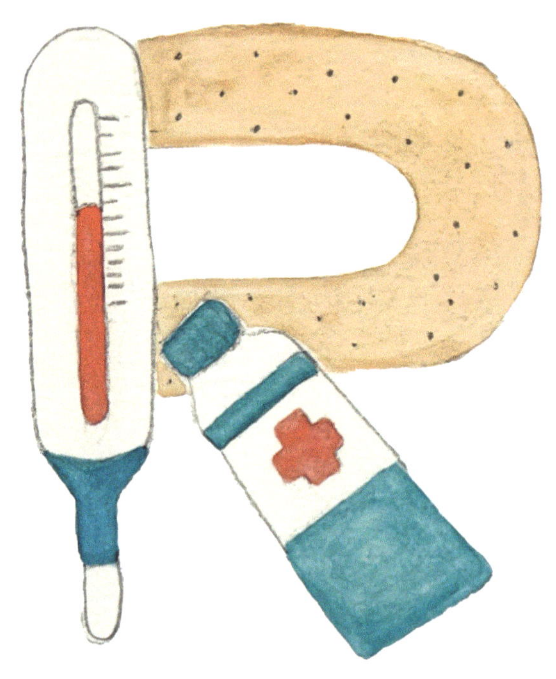

R is for Reaction.
If symptoms appear,
I know what to do and
keep my meds near.

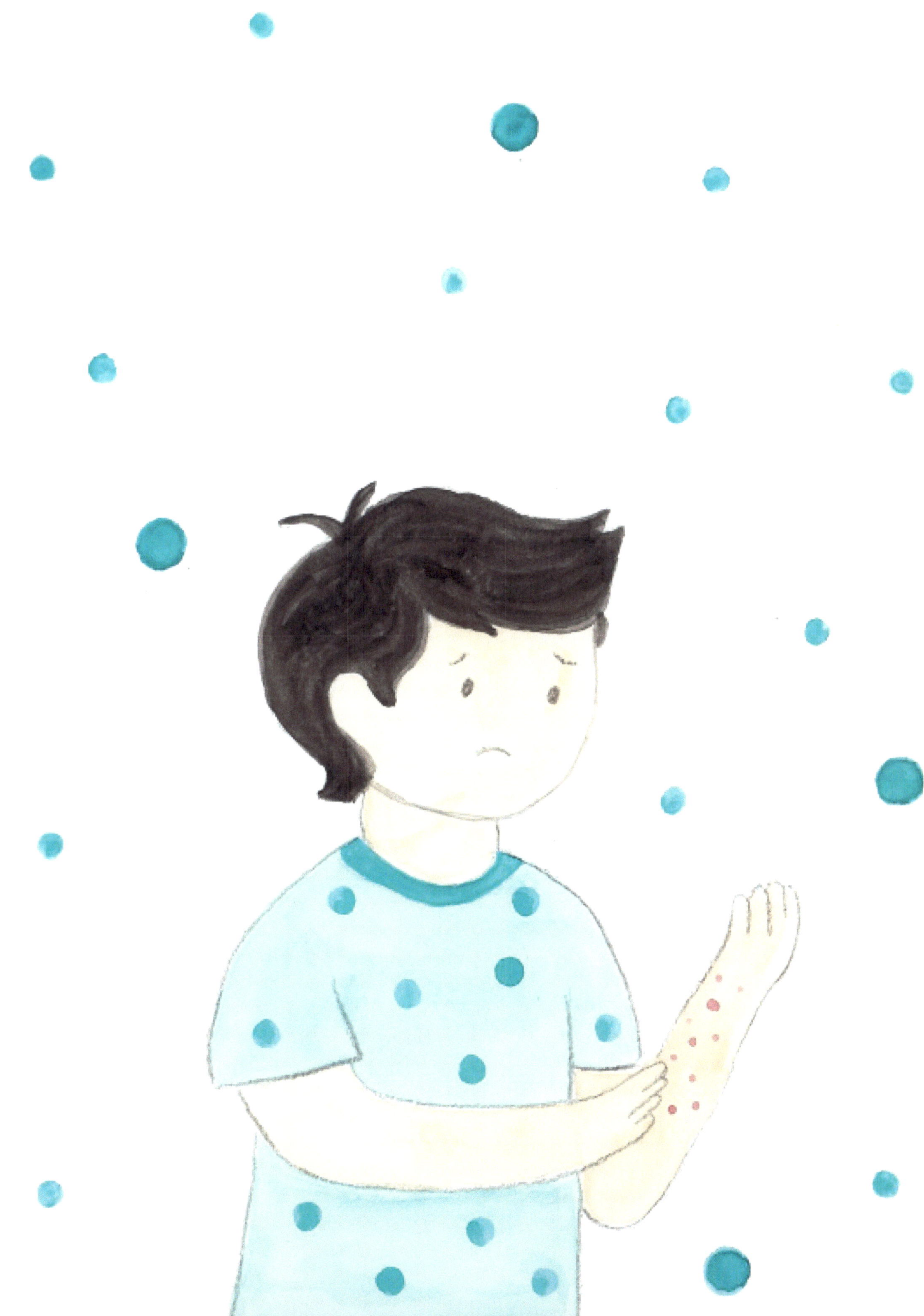

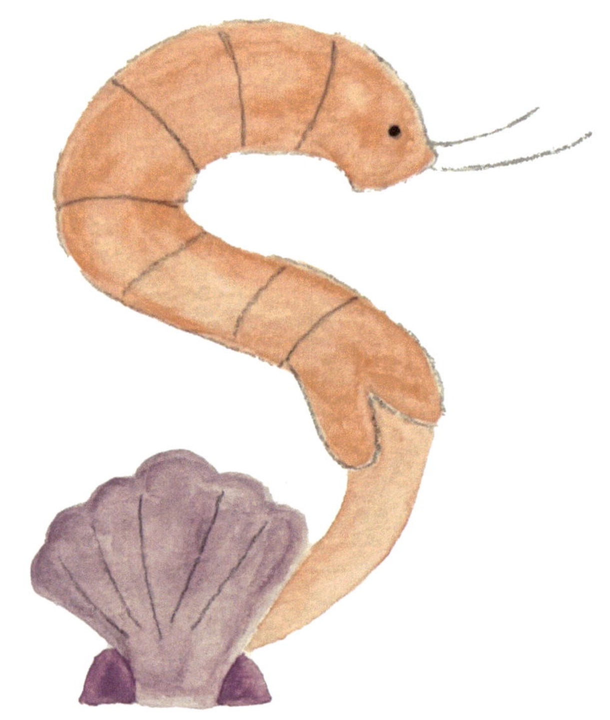

S is for Shellfish.
Shrimp, crabs, and clams,
if I eat them by mistake,
it causes a jam.

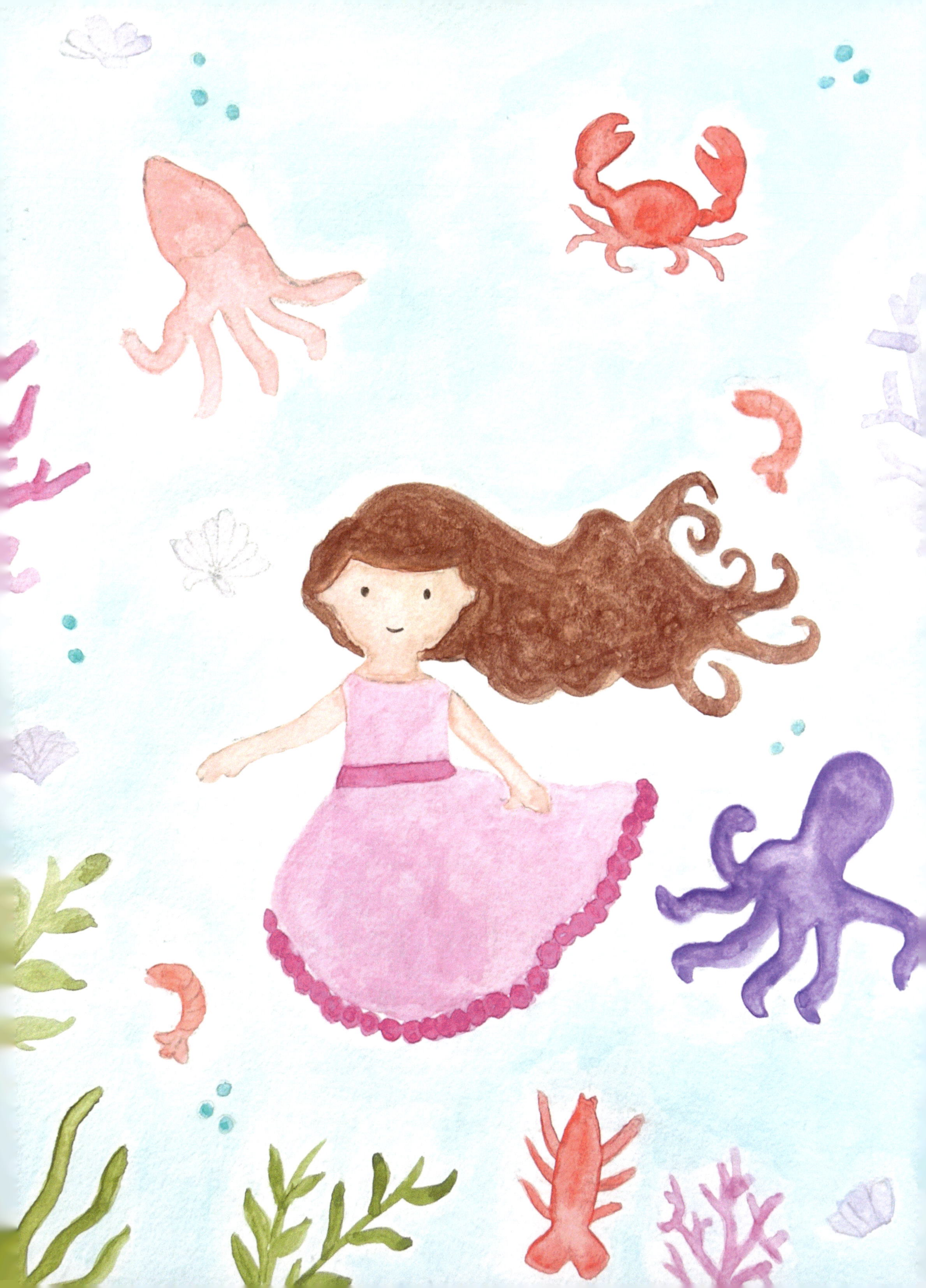

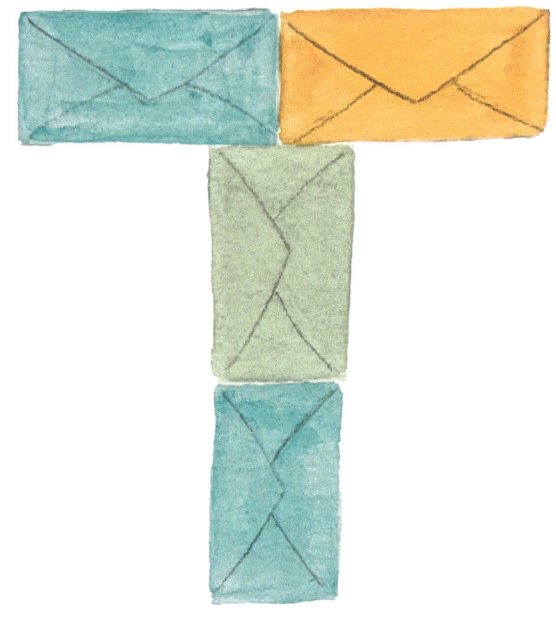

T is for Telling.
Don't wait or hide,
find someone you trust
and stand by their side.

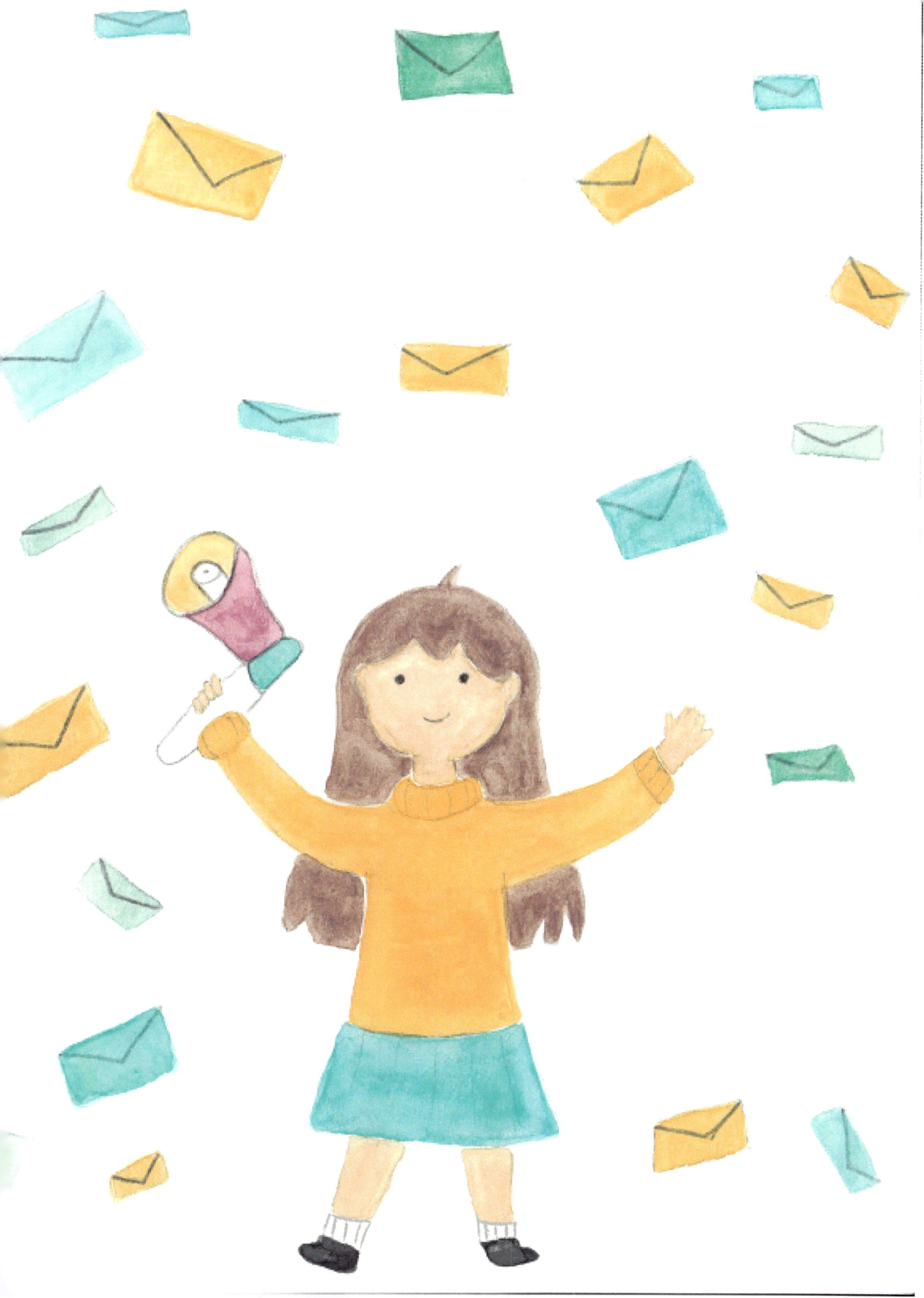

U is for Understanding.
Friends learn what to do
so everyone feels safe,
including you!

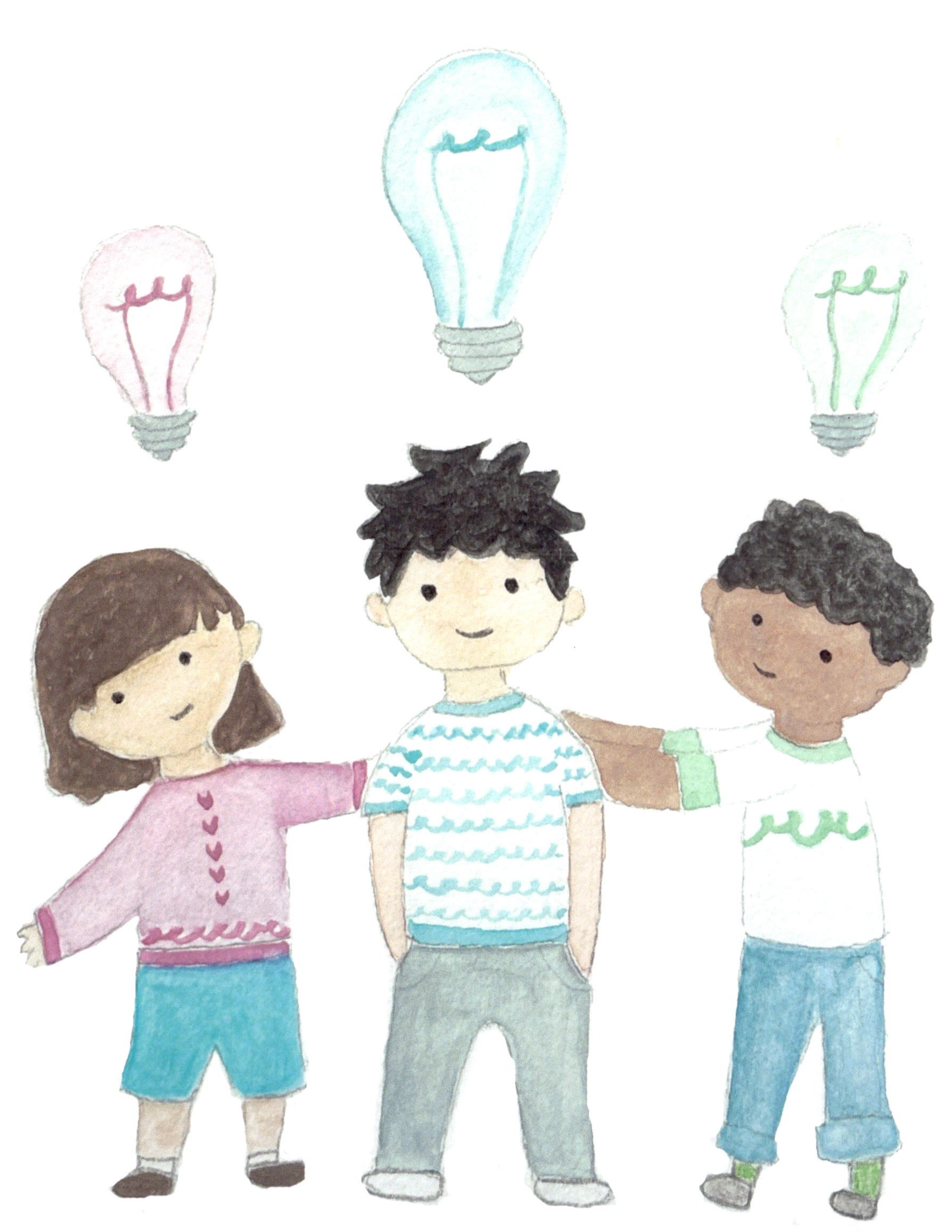

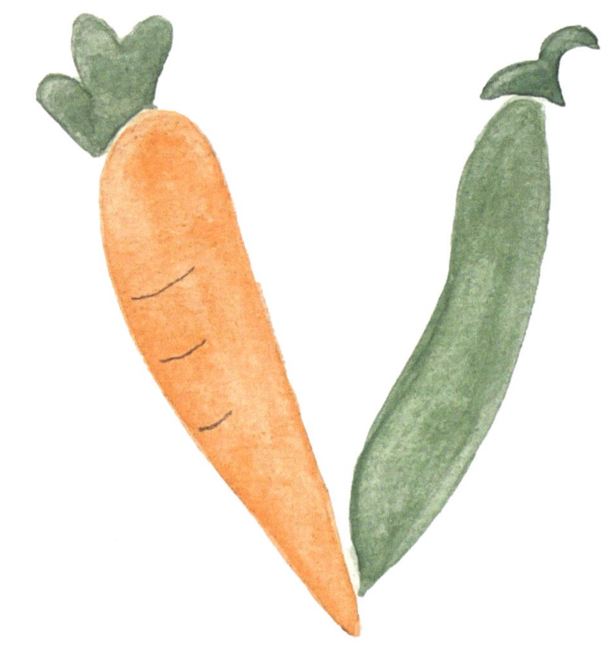

V is for Vegan.
It means no eggs, milk, or meat,
a friendly food choice
that's safe and sweet.

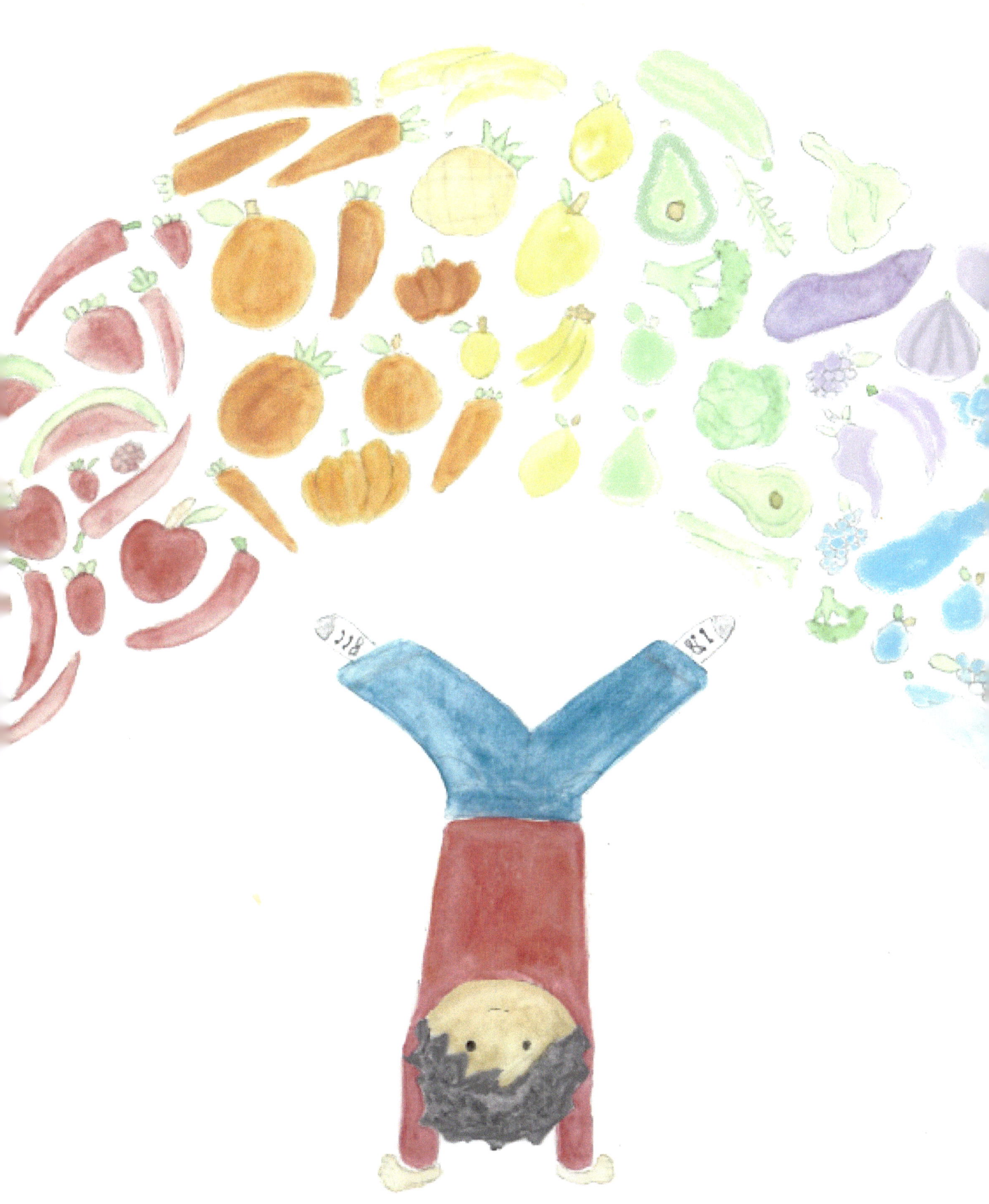

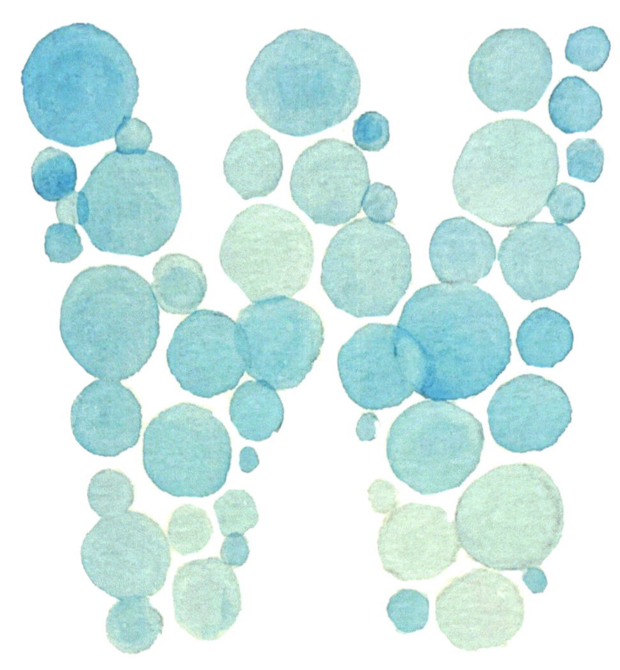

W is for Washing.
Before every bite,
everything's clean and
feels just right.

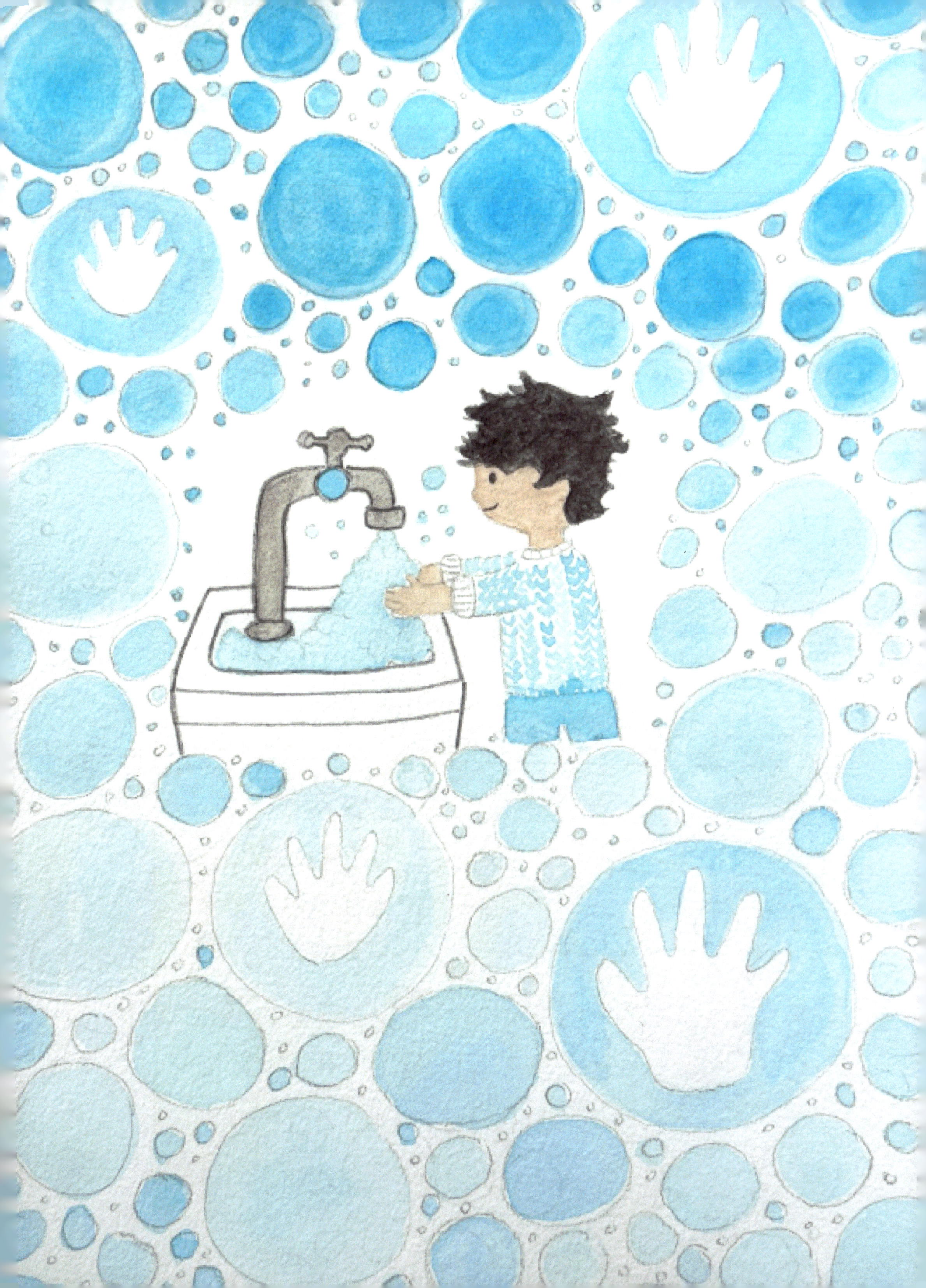

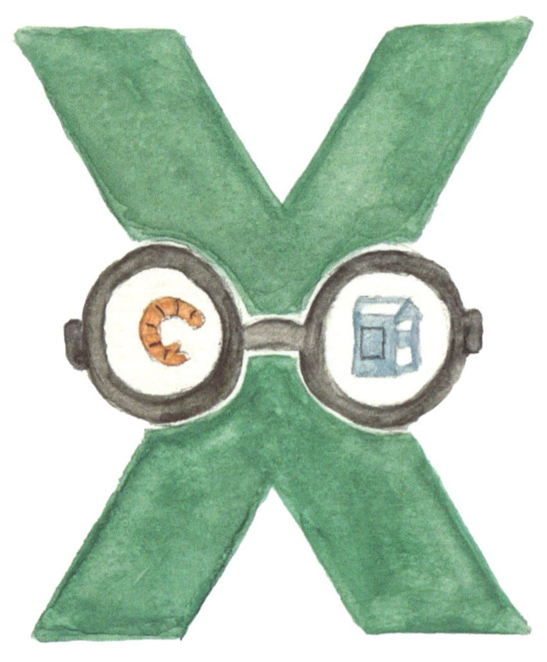

X is for X-Ray Vision.
We see what's inside,
to look for danger and
don't let it hide!

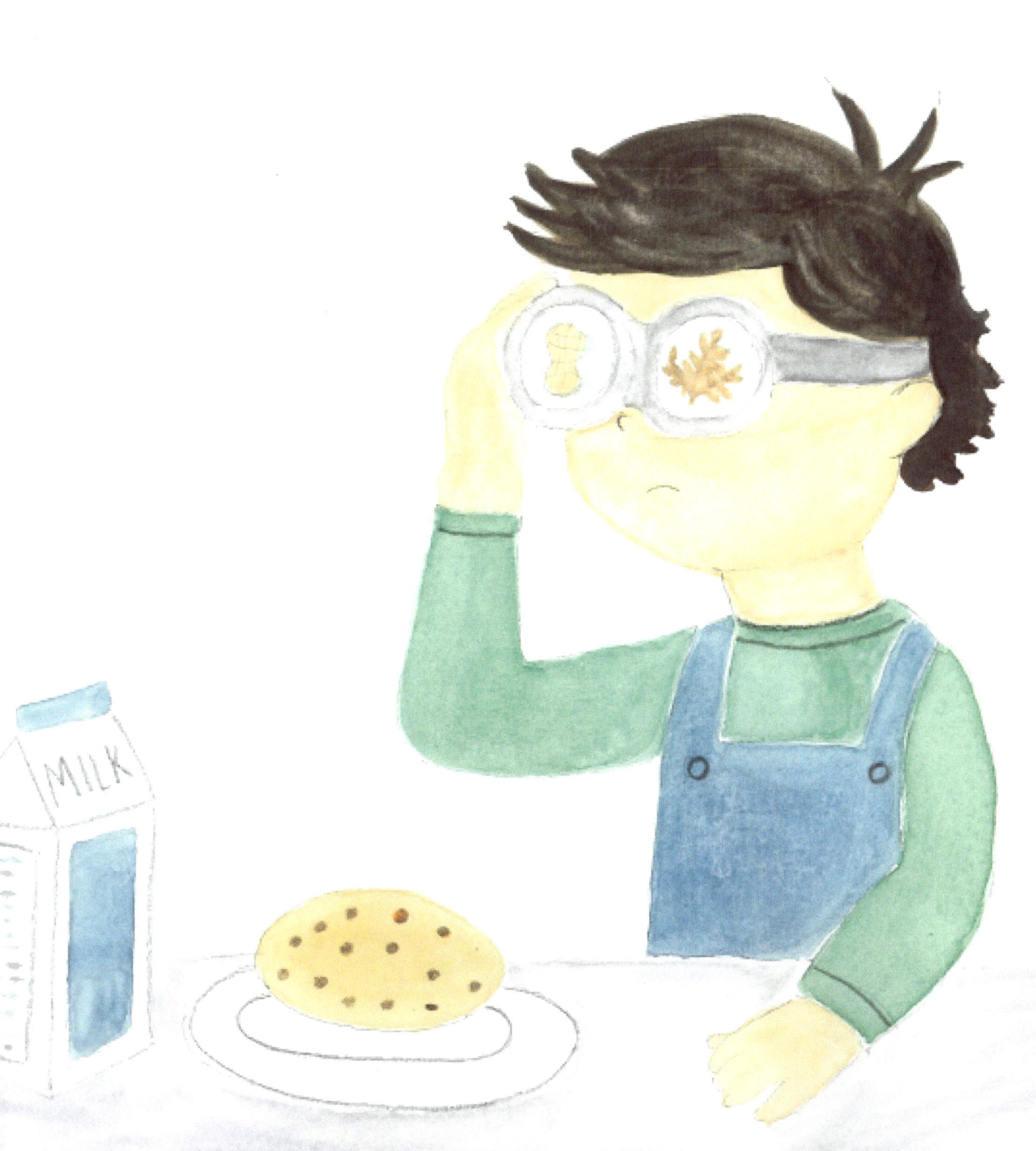

MILK

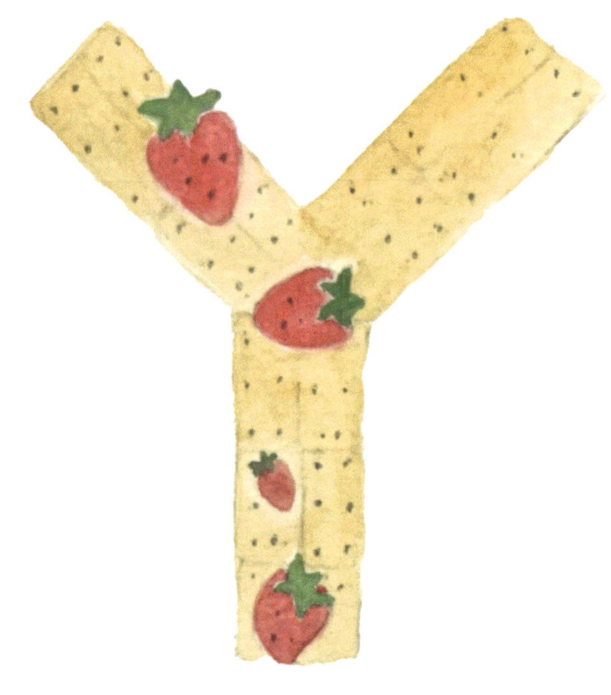

Y is for Yummy.
Safe treats we adore.
We don't feel left out,
we explore even more!

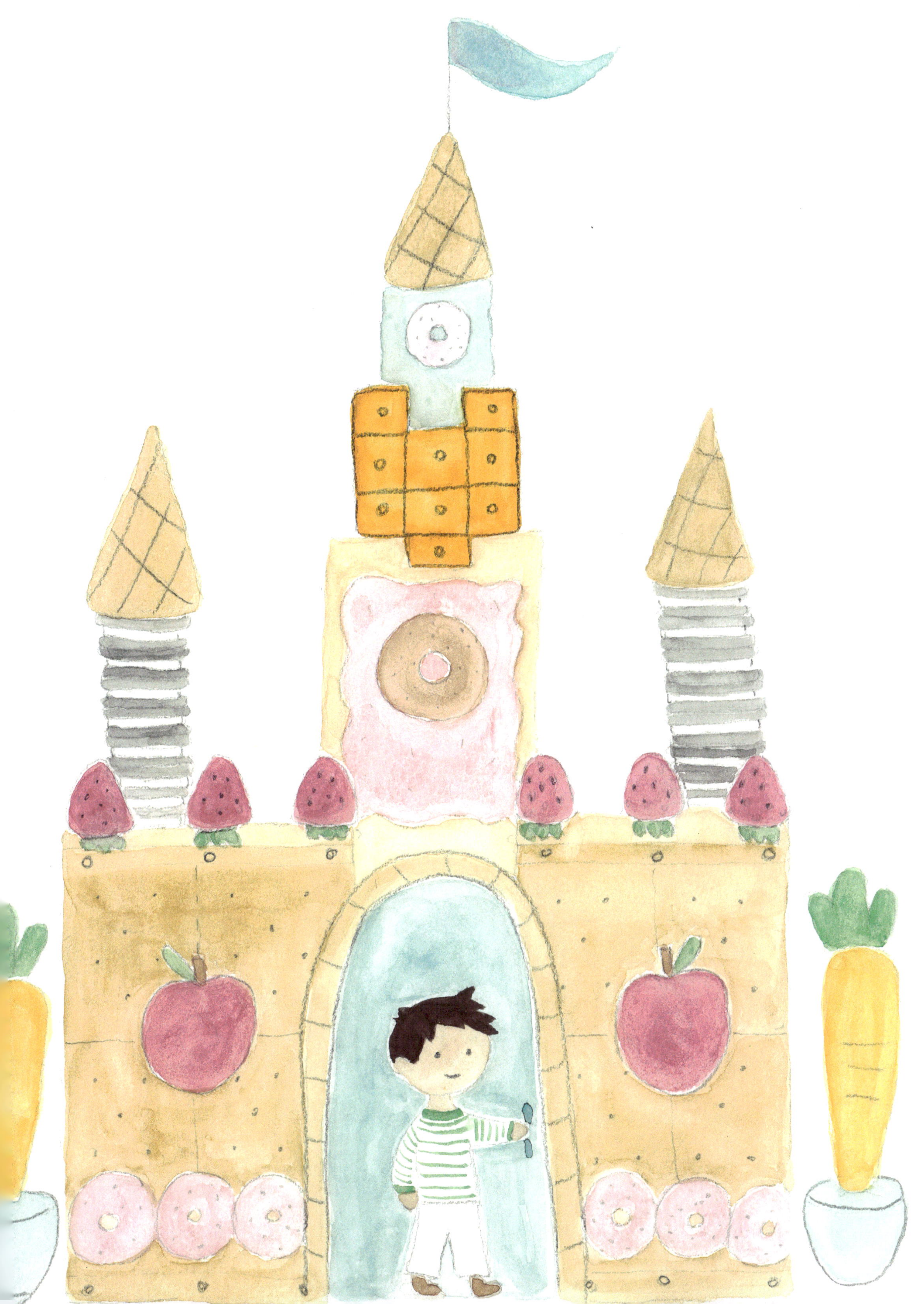

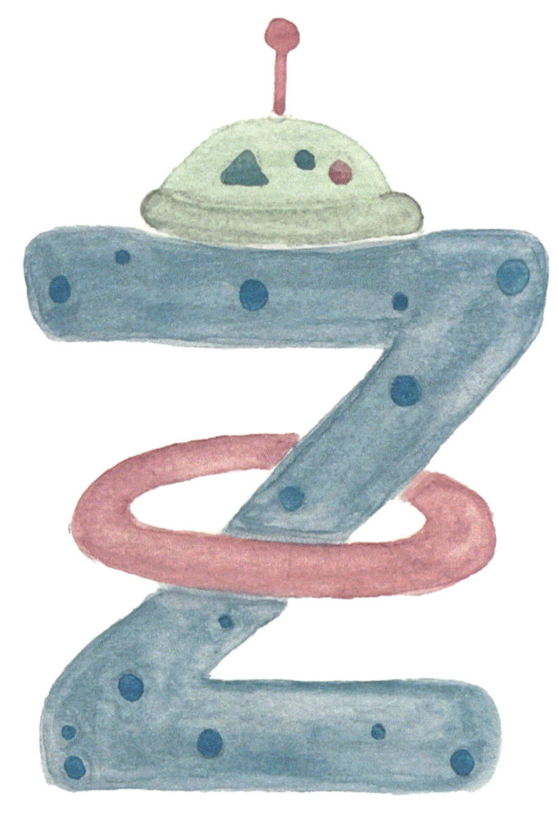

Z is for Zero Nut Zone.
Where snacks are safe
and friends can play,
we laugh and learn the
allergy-safe way.

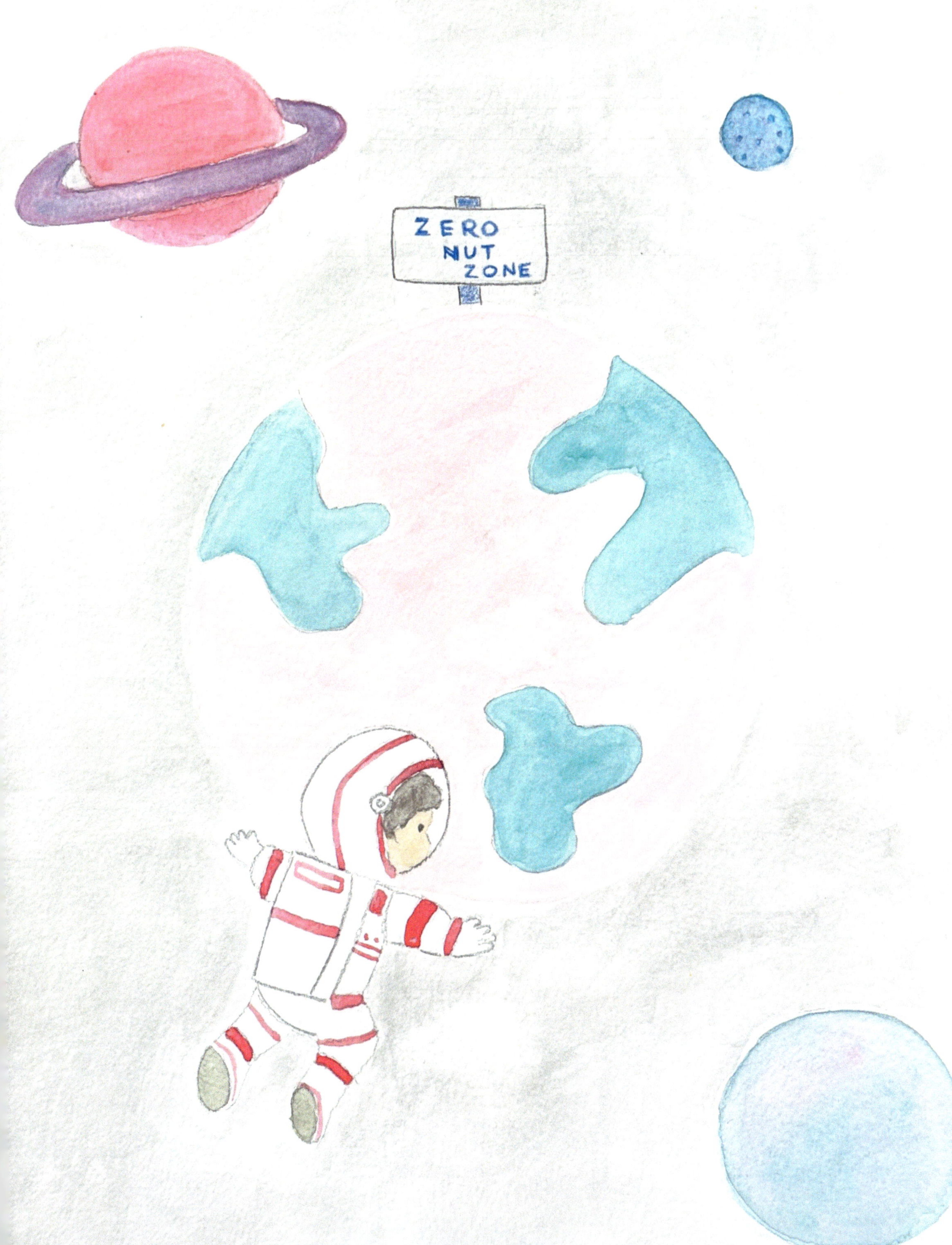

ZERO
NUT
ZONE

For The Grown-Ups

A short note parents, teachers, or caregivers:

This book is designed to empower young children to understand and navigate allergies with confidence and compassion. Whether a child has allergies or wants to support someone who does, these open the door for important conversations about safety, empathy, and self-advocacy.

The proceeds from this book go directly towards supporting allergy education and advocacy.

Thank you for helping us make the world a safer, kinder, more compassionate world for kids with allergies!

About the Author and Project

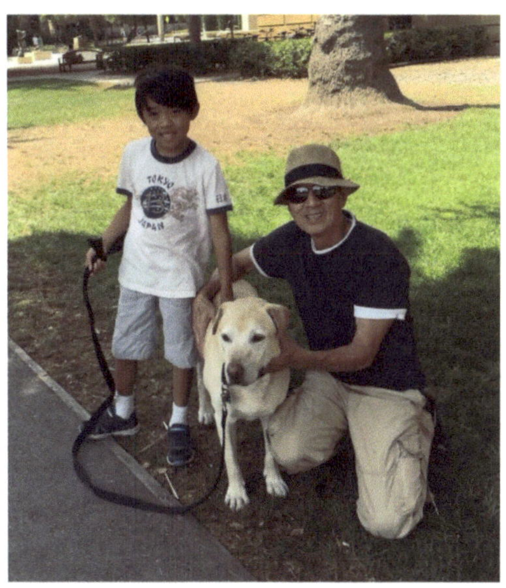

Maxwell Ngo is a high school student, artist, and allergy awareness advocate from Tustin, California. As someone who lives with a serious nut allergy, Max knows firsthand how scary and confusing food allergies can be, especially for young kids. That's why he created An Alphabet Allergy Adventure: Allergic to the Max, a fun and friendly way to teach kids and grown-ups how to stay safe, be kind, and understand allergies from A to Z.

When he's not writing or illustrating, Max enjoys playing soccer and volleyball, hanging out with family and friends, and volunteering in his community. He has received multiple national art awards, including from the Scholastic Art & Writing Awards, and was previously featured on ABC 7 and the Hallmark Channel for his inspiring hospital gown design for children.

Max and his friend Aayush Iyer are also 2025 Dragon Kim Foundation recipients, where they both received a grant to help raise awareness about food allergies. Max created this book hoping his story will empower kids to speak up, stay safe, and support their friends with allergies.